W9-AVZ-159

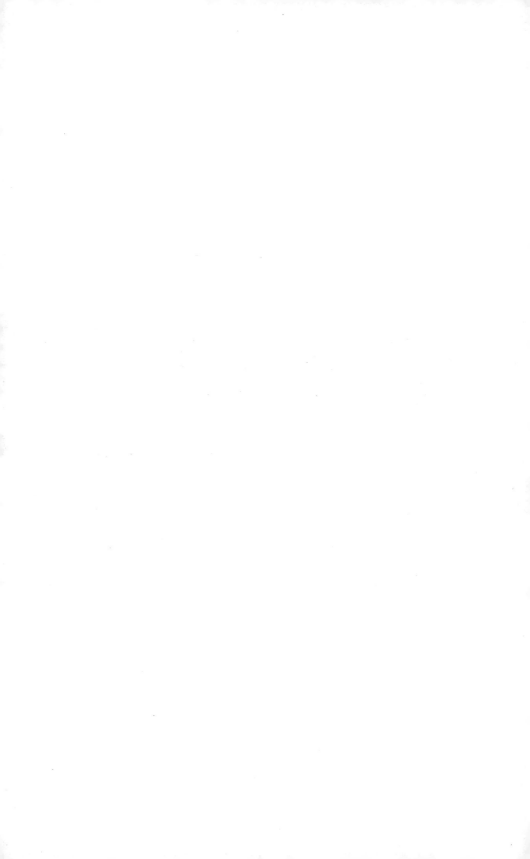

The Reading Glitch

How the Culture Wars Have Hijacked Reading Instruction— And What We Can Do About It

Lee Sherman
Betsy Ramsey

Rowman & Littlefield Education
Lanham, Maryland • Toronto • Oxford
2006

Published in the United States of America
by Rowman & Littlefield Education
A Division of Rowman & Littlefield Publishers, Inc.
A wholly owned subsidiary of The Rowman & Littlefield Publishing Group, Inc.
4501 Forbes Boulevard, Suite 200, Lanham, Maryland 20706
www.rowmaneducation.com

PO Box 317
Oxford
OX2 9RU, UK

Copyright © 2006 by Lee Sherman and Betsy Ramsey
Photographs by Paul Fardig and Judy Blankenship

All rights reserved. No part of this publication may be reproduced,
stored in a retrieval system, or transmitted in any form or by any
means, electronic, mechanical, photocopying, recording, or otherwise,
without the prior permission of the publisher.

British Library Cataloguing in Publication Information Available

Library of Congress Cataloging-in-Publication Data

Sherman, Lee, 1952–
  The reading glitch : how the culture wars have hijacked reading instruction—
and what we can do about it / Lee Sherman, Betsy Ramsey.
    p.   cm.
  Includes bibliographical references.
  ISBN-13: 978-1-57886-400-3 (hardcover : alk. paper)
  ISBN-10: 1-57886-400-3 (hardcover : alk. paper)
  ISBN-13: 978-1-57886-401-0 (pbk. : alk. paper)
  ISBN-10: 1-57886-401-1 (pbk. : alk. paper)
    1. Reading disability–United States.   2. Dyslexia–United States.   3. Effective
teaching–United States.   4. Reading–United States.   I. Ramsey, Betsy, 1949–
II. Title.
  LB1050.5.S456   2006
  371.91'44–dc22   2006004553

∞ ™ The paper used in this publication meets the minimum requirements of American
National Standard for Information Sciences—Permanence of Paper for Printed Library
Materials, ANSI/NISO Z39.48-1992. Manufactured in the United States of America.

For Dan and Jon,
whose courage is our inspiration

Contents

Acknowledgments   vii

Introduction   ix

1 Reading Disability: The Biological and Instructional Roots   1

2 The Reading Wars: Four Hundred Years of Stalemate   13

3 Collateral Damage: How Failed Reading Policies Hurt Kids   64

4 Bringing Reason to Reading: What Modern Science Reveals   116

5 Before Kids Fail: The Three Tiers of Prevention   162

6 It's Never Too Late: Rescuing Struggling Readers at Any Age   186

References   227

About the Authors   235

Acknowledgments

The heart and the soul of this book are the stories told here by teachers and tutors, principals and administrators, researchers and experts, parents and advocates, and, most of all, children and adults with dyslexia. Like a brush stroke on a van Gogh, each story contributes a daub of color to the canvas of reading disabilities. Blended together, they form a richly hued picture that we believe captures many essential truths about this complex subject. It is with deep gratitude that we acknowledge the commitment and the courage of Daniel Anderson, Chuck Arthur, Brian Baker, Barbara Bateman, Virginia Berninger, Debra Brooks, Jane Carter, Carl Cole, Dale, Roland Good, Jim Hanson, Dale Holloway, Ed Kame'enui, Kay Kaplan, Jeri Mackley, Alison Post, Jon Ruff, Chase Spittal, Kathy Spittal, Cindy Stadel, Carrie Swanson, Dan Tibbetts, "Tony," Dorothy Whitehead, William, Rhonda Wolter, Judy Wright, Cathy Wyrick, and Edie Wyrick.

Special thanks to Paul Fardig, not only for photographic excellence but for going the extra mile, and to Judy Blankenship for making images available for this project. Deep gratitude to Teri Sherman Matias for her generous contribution of graphic design, to Marcia Hilton for emergency reference services, and to Eugenia Potter, who introduced us to our editor Tom Koerner: Without you, Genia, this book would not exist.

We also wish to acknowledge the remarkable staff of the Bethel School District for creating a place where all children learn to read; the International Dyslexia Association (IDA); and especially the Oregon branch of the IDA for the educational opportunities, support, understanding, and friendships they have offered over many years and for their encouragement of research into the causes and remedies of dyslexia; Julie Anderson of the Oregon Department of Education for her dogged commitment to improving reading achievement for all kids and for her listening ear and her advice; and Diann Drummond of Portland Public Schools for being our mentor in all things special ed, and for encouraging our leadership and advocacy skills.

Thanks to Zack Anderson for tech support, to Mary Cutting for format troubleshooting, to Judy Fardig for photography assistance, to Joe Percival and James Sherman for strategic suggestions, and to Molly Falknor Percival for her endless love and support. Our thanks, too, to Patrick McGuire, Greg Meenahan, and Andree Cannon-Fleming of Thomas Edison High School in Portland, Oregon, for sharing their expertise with us. We also express our gratitude to kindergarten teacher Mary Lee Oshiro, who enlightened us with her years of hard-won wisdom.

We are most grateful for the expert transcription services of Patti Tucci and Lisa Wedge, without whom we would still be listening to tapes. And, finally, to our spouses Jim Anderson and Don Ruff, we express our loving appreciation for picking up the slack on the home front during the long months of research and writing, and for cheering us on.

PERMISSIONS ACKNOWLEDGMENTS

We gratefully acknowledge permission from Northwest Regional Educational Laboratory to reprint and to incorporate excerpts from previously published material:

Portions of several interviews from *Northwest Education*, 8(3), "The Hidden Disability," Spring 2003, have been reprinted here, along with excerpts from the editor's introductory column ("In This Issue" by Lee Sherman, p. 1), and the article ("Why Can't I Read?" by Lee Sherman, pp. 2–8).

Excerpts from the editor's introductory column ("Magic Chariot and Decoder Ring" by Lee Sherman, p. 1) from *Northwest Education*, 4(1), and "Succeeding at Reading," Fall 1998, have also been incorporated.

Introduction

The wooden staircase in my old grade school was slick and creaky. Damp leaves clung to my feet as I climbed. I wished desperately that Mom had let me buy the shoes I'd begged for at JC Penney, a slim, sophisticated pair of slip-ons in butter-soft leather. But instead of feeling sleek and graceful, as I imagined I would in the shoes Mom pronounced "impractical," I might as well have been one of those elephantine ballerinas in *Fantasia*, absurdly awkward-looking in their gauzy tutus. Clumping up the stairs with my feet buttoned into the fat rubber boots Dad made me wear to save my saddle shoes from the constant rains of north Seattle, I ached for invisibility. Keeping my head down and hugging the handrail, I held on to a fervent hope that I could duck into my classroom and shed the hated footwear before the boy I had a crush on noticed me.

The halls smelled like floor wax and bologna sandwiches and chalk dust. Kids' voices rang jarringly in the tunnel-like corridors, to which, periodically, the teachers would herd us for the bomb drills that were part of growing up during the Cold War. I remember lying on my stomach in my winter coat, my cheek pressed against the cold linoleum, my too-thin body sardined into a squirmy row of prostrate kids that stretched from front door to back door. With a stab of doubt, I wondered whether lacing my fingers behind my neck, as we were instructed, would really make me safe if Khrushchev dropped the A-bomb.

In this world that seemed so full of peril, I found a refuge. The school library, tucked away at the end of one dimly lit wing, was always warm from

ix

the steam that clanked in the heaters. The librarian welcomed students with an encouraging smile. Best of all, the shelves and shelves and shelves of books promised a million places to hide from put-downs about my stupid galoshes and rumors about Soviet nukes.

My strongest memories from those elementary years are, in fact, about books—ordering paperbacks from Scholastic, for instance. I would hungrily study the list of titles, wheedling Mom to let me order seven books instead of six—"Mom, just one more, *please!*" The day the books arrived was better than Christmas. I remember coming home one afternoon, holding my crisp new paperbacks covetously to my bony chest, and finding the house locked and empty. I felt scared and lonely for a minute or two, wondering what had happened to Mom who was always, always at home running the Hoover or cooking a ground-beef casserole. But then I thought of my books. Settling myself on the back porch in my pleated wool skirt and sensible shoes, I turned to chapter 1 of *Lad: A Dog*. The porch in suburban Seattle, bright with Mom's cherished geraniums, dropped away in an instant, and I was at Sunnybank in rural New Jersey at the turn of the last century.

Another time, I squirreled away a flashlight in my bedroom. After Mom said "sweet dreams" and flipped off the lamp, I waited till I knew she was settled next to Dad on the living-room sofa, watching the weekly episode of "Alfred Hitchcock Presents" or "The Untouchables," and then dug under my pillow for *Island of the Blue Dolphins*. Curled inside my cave of warm bedding, I read to the glow of the flashlight until I couldn't fight the heaviness in my eyes any more.

I remember Mrs. Bettinger as an assuring presence in my second-grade year, a year that I know now was critical to my future as a reader and as a student. Secure in her long seasons of experience, this grand matron managed her classroom with a firm set to her mouth but with friendly eyes that let you know there was a kind heart behind her no-nonsense focus on learning. Like practically every community in America, my suburban school system was using the Scott, Foresman and Co. "Dick and Jane" series of basal readers, based on a whole-word approach to reading; in essence, students memorized words by sight. But in Mrs. Bettinger's classroom, we also learned phonics. I don't know whether phonics instruction was mandated or merely tolerated in my school district. It may even have been flatly banned. My teacher might have been among the stealth "phonicators" you will read about in later pages of this book, who defied policy to give kids direct instruction in the alphabetic code.

Whether my phonics instruction was part of a larger curriculum or delivered by a master teacher on the sly, learning the rules—and, yes, the pesky exceptions—about the sounds of various combinations of letters and how those sounds blend to form words seemed like cool stuff to me, and very useful. I don't remember being bored by the instruction, ever. And contrary to the notion that phonics makes children cringe and cry, like getting a tooth filled, and that it makes them hate reading as much as they hate Brussels sprouts, phonics gave me the confidence to tackle tough books because I knew I could figure out any word at all. I wasn't limited to the words I had learned by sight, or even to the words in my spoken or heard vocabularies. I consciously used my phonics skills all the way through college, mentally breaking apart new, multisyllabic words, sounding them out, and adding them to my vocabulary.

When, as a writer new to the field of education, I began to hear the inflammatory talk about phonics instruction, I was puzzled. But having a lot of respect for my colleagues—many of them PhDs or EdDs—at a regional nonprofit, I figured I just had a lot to learn. I quickly gathered that the preferred method of teaching reading was called "whole language," and I immediately felt sure that this was the enlightened position. Wasn't it a great idea to deep-six those boring basals and, instead, immerse kids in the magical world of real stories? As a lifelong lover of literature, I was quite willing to accept this appealing notion.

But my easy acquiescence didn't last. A short while later when, as co-editor of *Northwest Education* magazine, I was putting together a series of articles on reading instruction, one of the PhDs in my organization insisted that I include information on "miscue analysis." That's when I encountered the "guessing" strategy taught in whole-language classrooms. It goes like this: When a young reader bumps into a word she doesn't know, the teacher tells her to look at the picture and think about what's happening in the story. "What word would make sense there?" the teacher prompts. Can't read it? Just guess. If you guess wrong, it's not a mistake, it's a "miscue." No problem. You'll get the gist of the story, if not all the fine points.

Here's how leading whole-language theorist Kenneth Goodman (1986) explains the process: "Readers predict, select, confirm, and self-correct as they seek to make sense of print. In other words, they guess or make hypotheses about what will occur in the text. Then they monitor their own reading to see whether they guessed right or need to correct themselves to keep making sense" (39).

A red flag the size of a Thanksgiving tablecloth unfurled in my mind that day. For me, the theory of whole language started to unravel. I was deeply troubled—horrified, really—to find out that every day in classrooms across America, hundreds of thousands of kids were being encouraged to guess as they learned to read. Research has revealed that contextual guessing is extraordinarily inaccurate. When those wrong guesses start to pile up as the child encounters more and more unfamiliar words in texts without picture clues, the meaning the child gleans is just a mushy approximation of what the author wrote. When the student gets to fourth grade and has to read for information—when the precise words are essential for grasping meaning—she will find herself lost in a miasma of unreadable words.

The statistics tell the story. Nationwide, only one-third of fourth-graders (32 percent) are able to read at grade level, according to the National Center for Education Statistics in 2003. Just one-fourth of them (24 percent) are proficient readers, and fewer than one in ten scores in the "advanced" range for reading. That leaves almost four in ten fourth-graders (37 percent) struggling along below the "basic" level.

The bedrock of whole language, as I came to learn, is the belief that printed language is as natural as spoken language. Learning to read, in this view, is instinctive, like learning to talk or walk. It follows that you could put a little kid in a roomful of books and nooks, read him wonderful stories, expose him to great literature, and he will become a reader in an osmosis-like way. And because he wasn't forced to focus on the mundane mechanics of print—such as how letters and sounds combine to form written words—he will grow up to love reading.

As a matter of fact, the "love of reading" gets a lot of discussion among whole-language advocates. The "need to read" gets hardly any. Prosaic tasks such as reading a bus schedule, a driver's test, a newspaper, a sign, a recipe, a set of instructions, a warning label, a prescription, a bank statement, or a tax form are ignored or taken for granted.

As someone who went through childhood and adolescence with my eyes glued to good books, I am a true believer in the power of literature to transmit culture, fuel imagination, incite wonder, and awaken passion. But most kids growing up in the United States will never know the formative and transforming power of the great works of great writers. That's because most schools' reading programs fail to give children the practical tools to tackle Tolstoy. But forget the great writers for a minute. Forget William Shakespeare and Maya Angelou and Arundhati Roy. Think instead about the most simple, day-to-day reading that carries us through the practical aspects of our lives. Far from being able to read classic novels like *War and Peace*, dramatic works like *Hamlet*, powerful poetry like *On the Pulse of Morning* (written for President Clinton's 1993 inauguration), or critically acclaimed novels such as Booker Prize winner *The God of Small Things,* countless Americans are defeated by even the lowliest level of survival reading. It's quite possible to live a productive and satisfying life without ever cracking a book deemed to have literary merit. But you'd better be able to read a food label, a job announcement, a computer manual, and a website.

The power that everyday, down-to-earth, just-figure-out-the-words reading holds over a life became heartbreakingly clear to us one day during an interview for this book. A young African American probationer we're calling "Tony" looked down at his hands, chagrined to admit that when he goes out to eat, he scopes out the restaurants beforehand. He chooses places with big, glossy menus featuring full-color photos of entrees and desserts. When you can't read the words for Tillamook cheeseburger or chicken Caesar salad or Chocolate Decadance, you live in fear of being found out by your dinner date. And when you can't read the phrases "roared their terrible roars" and "gnashed their terrible teeth," you make excuses when your five-year-old toddles up to you holding a copy of Maurice Sendak's *Where the Wild Things Are* and asks, "Daddy, will you read to me?"

The illusion that reading is "natural" is understandable. Some children take to reading as effortlessly as a fish takes to swimming. A few of these kids are savants. "He taught himself to read," their parents will say, at once proud and flummoxed. Other kids are blessed with an intuitive grasp of phonetic laws; give them a hint or two and off they go. But you can't explain the "instant" or "intuitive" reader by claiming that reading is an instinctive human behavior, any more than you can chalk up the gifts of golf phenom Ana Sorensen or software wizard Bill Gates to instinct. Some children have a knack for reading, just as some people have a knack for playing golf or designing software. But reading is no more "natural" than whacking a little white ball over a sand trap with a steel club. It's no more "instinctive" than creating 3-D graphics for hand-to-hand combat waged on a computer screen.

Whole language is a belief system whose fundamental assumption—that written language is embedded in our genes—is faulty. Written language, just like golf and software, is a human invention. English is based on an alphabetic code: This letter stands for this sound.

Writing encodes spoken language the same way sheet music encodes notes and rhythms. Humans across the planet have, for millennia, played drums and flutes, chanted, sung the songs of their ancestors. But the "natural" human ability to make music around a campfire doesn't segue automatically to playing written compositions by Bach or Schumann. Instead of "exposing" a child to music, the piano instructor teaches her student directly—which keys of ivory and ebony produce which notes, which combinations of keys produce which chords. She reveals to her student how to read the mysterious symbols that stand for A-sharp or B-flat in a process akin to matching sounds to letters. Many hours of practicing scales and exercises is the usual route to virtuosity. It's the rare individual who can play a sonata after simply attending a performance of the local chamber music ensemble.

Only when the musician is adept at reading the notes on the page is he free to play with joy and abandon, to interpret the compositions of great compos-ers, perhaps to write music of his own. This progression from basic skills to mastery is true of readers as well. In each case, a teacher passes along the collective knowledge of her discipline.

Researchers are showing us that adequate reading ability is attainable by every child when he or she is given the secret of print and taught to use it fluently. Studies show that it's not brain power but rather social standing (strongly linked to early literacy experience) that most often determines kids' quickness in catching on to the code. That's because in middle-class homes, the code is handed down from parent to child, like a family heirloom. With alphabet books, Mother Goose rhymes, and Dr. Seuss stories, affluent parents teach their children the letters and the sounds they stand for, just as they teach colors and shapes and the sounds that animals make. When these kids get to school and appear to learn reading in the whole-language classroom, the teacher says, "See, it works." But as prominent researcher Reid Lyon, for-merly of the National Institutes of Health, scoffs, "any cockamamie approach" will seem to work with these kids.

The ugly reality is that whole-language instruction, which skips over skills in a rush to meaning, favors kids who have this literary lineage. As a number of researchers have observed, whole language is best suited for the children of the educated classes. Whole-language proponents argue that children will be bored by tedious rules about sounds and spelling. They will be turned off, maybe even hate books. So the method essentially "starts in the middle." This can work nicely for kids who bring a lot of advance knowledge to school.

But kids who don't know Dr. Seuss from Dr. Dre, or Mother Goose from Queen Latifah, are left behind. For them, the secrets of written language remain hidden, inscrutable, mysterious, alien. Most likely, their parents never received the code, either. And so, by tailoring teaching to the children of edu-cated parents, schools have spawned an insidious elitism that, over time, has hardened into intergenerational poverty—essentially, a caste system.

When schools hold back the code, no matter how pure the motive, no mat-ter how lofty the theory, they deprive students of full participation in the world. No one argues with the obvious fact that parents are children's first teachers. But if parents, for reasons of illiteracy, poverty, or family dysfunc-tion, fail to fulfill the role well, many educators say, "It's a shame that these kids are unprepared." Hardly anyone would take on the hugely demanding, largely undervalued job of teaching unless he or she cared a lot about kids—the ones who qualify for free school lunches as well as the ones who bring turkey breast on oat bran in their insulated tote bags. But the U.S. educational system is permeated with a stubborn conviction that, in the end, you can't really expect much of kids who have poorly educated parents. And so, without meaning to, these educators help perpetuate the cycle of poverty in America.

"Well, if teachers are falling short with at-risk kids, it's not for a lack of commitment," observes my spouse, Jim Anderson, who teaches middle school in a rough section of town nicknamed "Felony Flats" because so many of the locals are in and out of prison for drugs and other crimes. Every afternoon he sees his colleagues, weighted down with pounds and pounds of student assignments, heading home for an evening of grading essays and term reports. "They care *so much*," Jim says.

Despite those teachers' dogged determination, nearly 60 percent of the eighth-graders at Lane Middle School are falling short of state benchmarks in reading. Yet in the leafy hills across town, students at West Sylvan Middle School—the privileged sons and daughters of the professional class—earn reading scores that look like Lane's turned upside-down. At this elite school (where it was once rumored that girls could join the "Hundred-Dollar Club" if each day's outfit had a big enough price tag), 90 percent of eighth-graders are reading at benchmark. In fact, nearly 65 percent of West Sylvan's students are *exceeding* state standards in reading. Down on the Flats, only 10 percent of Lane's eighth-graders achieved an "exceeds benchmark" score in 2003–2004.

The common wisdom says, "Poor kids can't be expected to read at levels comparable to those of rich kids." Researchers respond by answering: "Yes, they can, if they get science-based reading instruction, beginning on Day 1 of kindergarten and continuing throughout secondary school."

The other big category of kids typically left out of the readership clique are those who have a brain glitch—a biologically based reading disability that requires intensive, systematic instruction to overcome. If explicit code instruction is critical for just about every young reader, it is even more essential for children with dyslexia. That's because language deficits go deepest for them. The authors of *The Scientist in the Crib*, Alison Gopnik, Andrew Meltzoff, and Patricia Kuhl, make the vital point that "in order to read and write, you have to translate the system of language sounds directly into a system of written letters" (1999, 121). The typical kid with a reading disability has enormous trouble with sounds as well as with print, failing to hear the distinctions between letters such as *r* and *l*, or *b* and *p*. Subtle as those distinctions are, most of us could hear them at birth, the researchers explain.

When I first met nine-year-old Daniel, before his disability was diagnosed, I noticed that his large vocabulary was riddled with mispronunciations—*ak lease* for *at least, pellow* for *pillow, whooped* instead of *whipped* cream. Even as he received intensive help in middle school, he continued to mis-hear common words. For example, he would complain about his eleven o'clock *curse-you* (for "curfew"), or recount a story about someone who committed *sewer-side* (for "suicide"). His creative mispronunciations are funny sometimes, but the hard reality is that his problems with sound-letter mapping will make his reading a chore forever.

Research has shown again and again that all children, including the disadvantaged and the learning disabled, *can* learn to read adequately when given direct, explicit, systematic instruction in phonics. Despite countless studies that affirm this, however, the whole-language philosophy shuns phonics, demonizing it as a right-wing plot against progressive teaching methods.

If you advocate phonics, whole-language proponents brand you as a religious fundamentalist and/or a radical conservative. They figure you must be against reproductive choice for women, sex ed for teens, and equal rights for gays. Your pro-phonics stance makes you a likely card-carrying member of the National Rifle Association who thinks students ought to start their day with a prayer, learn creationism alongside evolution, and eat in a cafeteria where the Ten Commandments are posted in bold type above the lunch line. You're probably even guilty of questioning the sexual orientation of cartoon characters like SpongeBob SquarePants and Tinky Winky.

This politicization of phonics has rendered the national conversation about reading instruction nasty, shrill, and impervious to reason and science.

I once asked a principal and bush pilot in Alaska to explain his fondness for direct instruction, which at his charter school included lessons in Latin and Greek roots. He threw a question back at me. "Can you teach someone to fly a jet by simply *exposing* them to a Boeing 747?" The derision in his voice was withering. Here's another question: Can you prepare an aspiring astronaut for a lunar mission by simply letting her hang around NASA? As renowned reading researcher Louisa Cook Moats argues, reading *is* rocket science and should be taught with the same kind of rigor.

There are millions of reasons to do this. Each of those reasons has a name and a face and a future that in large measure hinges on reading. One of those reasons is my nephew Keenan, a Cambodian orphan who came to live with my sister and her husband at twenty months of age. "Busy and clever" were the adjectives that accompanied his first snapshots from the orphanage. The tiny child with the thousand-watt smile has lived up to both descriptors every minute he's been in our family. A few weeks ago, Keenan turned four. Relishing his new status as a big kid, he told me, "Auntie Lani, when I'm five I'm going to be in kindergarten, and when I'm six, I'm going to go to first grade and learn how to *read*!"

—Lee Sherman
April 2005

II

For decades, reading disability was considered a moral failing of the individual: The kid's just not trying. He could do better if only he worked harder. He *must* be lazy because he's certainly bright enough—brighter, in fact, than a lot of his buddies who seem to read pretty well. The other popular theory is a deficit in the family—a failing of parental skill or intelligence or background or income. Another notion crops up, too: that overachieving middle-class parents just can't accept their child's intellectual limitations, so they make excuses and demand special-ed services. Even today, amidst the explosion of evidence supporting a biological basis for learning disabilities, plenty of well-meaning educators continue to blame children and their parents for the glitch in the print-processing part of their brain.

The irony is that kids with dyslexia are actually working harder than anybody else because of the way the circuits in their brains are wired. We know this because researchers at Yale and the University of Washington have taken images of readers' brains at work. Yet educational practice, tragically for millions of kids, lags years behind the science.

Reading disability only matters in a print-based culture. In a hunter-gatherer society, the skill set for success has nothing to do with deciphering words encrypted in print. Speed and stealth, tracking ability and true aim, a powerful throwing arm, a gift for crafting arrows and bows, a sixth sense about animal behavior and habitat—these are the abilities a hunter needs to survive and thrive. My dyslexic son Jon, for whom reading continues to be a mighty struggle, could well have been a prodigy in a different kind of culture in another place and time, where his unique patterns of thinking—his observational powers, intuitive gifts, auditory learning skills—would be highly adaptive.

I often ask people to think about this scenario: What if music—singing on key—were the skill you needed to be successful in life? If carrying a tune were the standard, how many of us would be collecting cans instead of collecting a paycheck? Musical ability is just another set of neurological skills that some people come by naturally. Fortunately for the tone deaf among us, hardly anyone has to sing an aria to get a job.

As the twentieth century wound down, reading rose on a steep trajectory to claim a central position in success—from a luxury of the elite, college-educated class to a fundamental activity of just about any workplace. While educators argue about the best way to teach reading—debating the definition of "real reading," trading political and ideological barbs, spitting verbal venom—millions of children fail to learn this most critical of life skills.

Meanwhile, at universities from coast to coast, researchers have fomented a quiet revolution. I've closely followed the work of renowned scientists and educators such as Sally and Bennett Shaywitz at Yale, Joseph Torgesen at Florida State University, and Edward Kame'enui at the University of Oregon for years. Those of us who have watched our children struggle are deeply heartened to have top-notch scientists and research-savvy advocates informing the public that reading disability is not a moral failing of smart children and their parents, but a difference in how their brains work. The light that thirty-plus years of National Institutes of Health research—spanning administrations both conservative and liberal, Republican and Democrat—has directed on the science behind our understanding of dyslexia ought to be illuminating the work of teachers in classrooms everywhere.

Yet Sally Shaywitz, at a symposium on brain research in Eugene, Oregon, in the late spring of 2004, expressed profound frustration at the failure of the education community to embrace the findings of this rigorous science emanating from some of our most elite universities. "The puzzle is beginning to come together because of the convergence of research," she said, looking almost beseechingly at the scattered audience. "This convergence of evidence heralds the possibility of a new era in education. The frustration is that in any other field, this information would be grabbed up so quickly. But it's happening so slowly in education."

As a longtime researcher designing and performing biochemical experiments in the Oregon Cancer Institute at Oregon Health and Science University, I struggle daily with how to translate solid research evidence into clinical use. My work in breast cancer studies—certainly an area of extreme import and urgency—has taught me how agonizingly slow the research-to-practice process proceeds in the field of medicine. But it is even more agonizing to see the glacial pace at which research knowledge creeps into classroom application in the field of education.

The lives wasted as children are subjected to classroom malpractice should be of imminent concern to pediatricians and teachers, as they are to the distraught parents of kids who fail to read. Yet too many teachers are impeded by dangerous ideologies and baseless beliefs about reading instruction that block reason and encumber progress. And too many physicians are held back by outdated notions, such as the idea that dyslexics suffer from a visual disorder causing them to see backwards, long discredited yet still widely believed. Medical schools need to better prepare future pediatricians to identify learning disabilities in their patients and to give advice on how to treat them. Practitioners in both education and medicine need more understanding about the important differences and relationships between attention deficit disorder and dyslexia.

Because so many educators, doctors, and parents either miss the clues or lack the facts, most dyslexic kids aren't identified till third, fourth, or fifth grade. That's too late. The research shows that kids who are not reading by third grade almost never catch up. And the later the intervention, the greater the emotional damage. There are basically two kinds of kids: those whose disruptive behavior calls attention to a reading problem and those who fake their way through—the kids who act out tend to get extra help sooner. A lot of other kids, especially girls, will stay off the teacher's radar by being cooperative and relying on their strengths—such as finely honed auditory learning abilities—to fool teachers, classmates, and even parents.

Our hope with this book is to present researchers and science-driven practitioners in a human and approachable way so that educators see that an interdisciplinary approach to helping children with learning disabilities will produce the best results. Scientists, educators, and parents are all working in the field because they are committed to children and want the best for them. We offer this book as another perspective on the philosophical hostilities that have divided educators in Europe and America, literally for centuries. We believe that by embracing science, classroom teachers can help lead their craft to new levels of professionalism—and children to new levels of achievement.

The other day, my dyslexic son Jon, a recent graduate of the University of Oregon, commented that although we've come a long way, we still have lots to learn about the biological underpinnings of dyslexia. We look forward to the work that teases out the details of what we in cancer research call the "genomic" (having to do with chromosomes and genes and DNA) and "proteonomic" (having to do with proteins that are the expression of the gene code) constructs in the next decades. In the meantime, Jon wants me to enroll in Orton-Gillingham tutor training so I'll be able to teach his children to read when they come along, because they may well inherit their father's brain glitch. He figures we may still be waiting for the schools to catch up.

—Betsy Ramsey
April 2005

Reading Disability: The Biological and Instructional Roots

Little kids are tender individuals, easily frustrated and ashamed of deficient reading skills once they notice that many of their classmates read so effortlessly.

—G. Reid Lyon, *Washington Post*, 1996

We now know that dyslexia affects one out of every five children—ten million children in America alone. . . . Once a pattern of reading failure sets in, many children become defeated, lose interest in reading, and develop what often evolves into a lifelong loss of their own sense of self-worth.

—Sally Shaywitz, *Overcoming Dyslexia*, 2003

The new teacher was alarmed to discover that so many of his third-graders were hapless readers, stymied by the written word. But he was certain that wonderful stories, engagingly told, could unlock the mysteries of print for any child. So he lavished upon his students the riches of literature, steeped them in the magic of good books. When June rolled around, however, he was dismayed to find that the same children who could barely read in September—fully one-third of the class—were no less lost as they headed home for summer break.

"Their reading remained slow and effortful, the time it took to read text was so great that they could not remember what they read, and their spelling was still lousy," the teacher recalled several decades later. "The only change I could discern was that their motivation to learn had waned, and their self-esteem had suffered substantially."

The teacher felt he had failed his young charges. He abandoned the classroom—but not the profession. For a decade and a half, he was a driving force for science-based interventions for struggling readers across America.

G. Reid Lyon, who was chief of the branch of the National Institutes of Health that sponsored studies on reading from the early 1990s until 2005, told the above story to Congress in 2000 as he made a case for more and better research on how kids learn to read and why so many bright children can't crack the code. The big challenges, he said, are twofold: one, to unravel the secrets of learning disabilities that keep kids shut out of literacy; and two, to overcome those disabilities with proven interventions. In a world driven by the written word, the damage done by untreated reading problems can be devastating—to kids, to families, to society.

"Reading disability is not only an educational problem," Lyon wrote in the *Washington Post* in 1996, "it is a major public health and economic concern" (1996b, R18).

THE STORY OF JON, AS TOLD BY BETSY RAMSEY

People were packed into the front room of our big old house, and they were starting to seep into the kitchen—aunts and uncles and neighbors, friends of a lifetime, and an ebullient bunch of college kids. We were celebrating my son's graduation from the University of Oregon. The lump lodged in my throat was the physical manifestation of the knot of feelings knocking around inside me—pride, of course, and relief, and something dreamlike: Is this really happening? I was an emotional jellyfish.

But Jon had the look of a person who's completely comfortable in his own skin as he shambled into the kitchen to grab a beer from the ice chest and then, with an understated sense of humor and a cool slouch of the shoulders, held court with his buddies. A newcomer to his life wouldn't guess that there had been a time when no one could have foreseen this day.

It was twenty-two years ago that I held this child, a warm bundle of squalling potential, in my arms at Portland's Kaiser Hospital. What I never could have imagined on that first day of Jonathan's life was that my bright-eyed firstborn would lead me to a lifetime of advocacy for kids with learning disabilities.

At first, everything seemed fine in our green-and-white Craftsman-style home in one of Portland's solid, inner-city neighborhoods. My half-time job in cancer research left me lots of time to dote on my child. His engineer father, though a little dazed with the duties of parenthood, was as devoted a dad as you could find. As Jonathan grew and crawled and toddled, he was

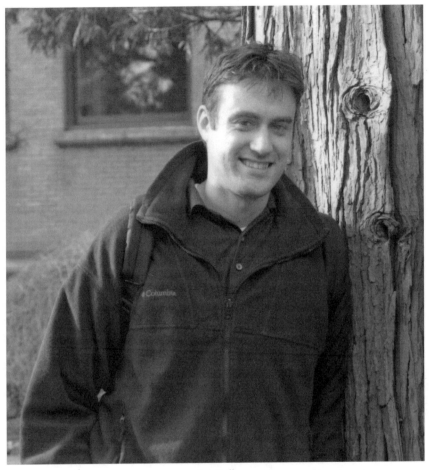

Jon Ruff

smart and funny and busy—and very, very sociable. From those very first years, he preferred playing with other kids to playing with toys.

At the end of every day, as he burrowed into his pillow under a pile of warm covers, he would listen intently to the fairy tales and nursery rhymes his dad or I would read to him. His favorite was an alphabet book about the sounds that animals make. He knew every sound by heart and always gave an especially enthusiastic rendition of *cock-a-doodle-do*! He never, ever went to sleep without a bedtime story to take to his dreams.

We had no reason to suspect a problem.

It wasn't until he was five that we started to worry. Despite an all-day, enriched preschool program, his prereading skills were just about nil on the day we dropped him off for his first day of kindergarten. He hit a wall right away: trying to write his eight-letter name. To make it easier, we lopped off some letters and started to call him Jon. (Later, when his letters and words were all coming out backward, our family joke was to call him "Noj.") Mid-year, he scored in the 17th percentile on an assessment. Our level of concern rose another notch. I told his teacher that my husband and I had a couple of college degrees apiece and we were pretty sure Jon should be at least average. She reassured us with an indulgent smile: "He'll catch up. He's just not ready to read."

But by the end of his first-grade year in a dual-language Spanish immersion program, our little boy still couldn't make sense of print. Reading eluded him well into second grade, and the emotional turmoil was boiling over into our home life. Jon's near-daily tantrums and fits over schoolwork were out of character for this kid who had always before been good-natured and happy. At our insistence, the school placed him in a resource room for one hour, twice a week, for help overcoming what they termed vaguely as a "specific learning disability."

When your child is born with a learning disability, it's hidden at first. He has all ten fingers and toes, and sparkling eyes. He walks at the right age and talks at the right age. All of a sudden, you have to confront this new reality. Jon's dad and I had to make a radical shift in our thinking. We had to accept what seemed impossible: Our smart little boy needed—would always need—special help with learning.

Resigned but resolute, we set about to help our child grow as far and as fully as his potential would allow. In our case, as in so many cases of learning disability, that potential turned out to be far, far greater than we could imagine at the moment of diagnosis. All we could see then were the daunting hurdles that stood in his way.

Knowing next to nothing about learning disabilities, we checked around and decided to get an independent assessment from a private, nonprofit group of specially trained tutors. A specialist at Language Skills Therapy gave us a more precise diagnosis than the school had offered: Jon, she said, had dyslexia. We'd barely ever heard the term, much less a definition. His disability, she told us, was moderately severe. She said he needed specific instruction in reading, writing, spelling, and math—daily.

The resource room wasn't nearly enough to help Jon catch up and keep up. But in those days, we didn't know enough about special-education laws to argue with the school that he should have more than he was getting. The worst day of our lives as parents was the day we sat down with Jon's third-grade teacher for the routine parent-teacher conference and asked, "How's he doing?" The teacher said, encouragingly, "He's doing pretty well—he's not crying every day like he did at the beginning of the year."

We hired a tutor. For the next four years, she worked with Jon for an hour after school, three days a week. I tried to stay in the background, hanging out in the kitchen listening to the news on National Public Radio. But I couldn't resist turning down the volume, just a little, and peering between the swinging doors into the dining room to eavesdrop on the lessons. The tutor, who was trained in the multisensory technique called Orton-Gillingham, led Jon through the letters and sounds, integrating writing with speaking, reading with spelling. Each lesson ended with oral reading from literature: She would read a sentence, then Jon would read a sentence. They would discuss vocabulary and the story as it unfolded—the setting and plot, characters and climax.

Jon never once moaned or griped, despite missing out on after-school romps with his pals. He was, at last, learning to read. "Everyone else was playing on Big Wheels," he recalled recently, a little wistfully. "But the tutoring made me feel like I was smarter."

We joined a support group at Lewis & Clark College for LD kids and their families. It's called Reversals—a word play on the common phenomenon among dyslexics of writing letters backwards. There, we learned about the law—the Individuals with Disabilities Education Act—and the things you need to do to be a good parent of an LD child. We learned that Jon *could* succeed and go to college.

Meanwhile, I read to him every night all the way through middle school—his textbooks, his literature assignments, his personal reading. The mysterious and the supernatural were his genres of choice—creepy ghost stories, sightings of the Loch Ness monster, rumors of Bigfoot lurking in the Northwest's fabled old-growth forests. Against my own inclinations, I became an expert in Sasquatch.

We got books on tape from the Oregon State Library for the Blind. I would check out the print version at the county library, and Jon would read along with the tape. It improved his vocabulary, syntax, and fluency. We had a Spanish-speaking friend who read his Spanish-immersion textbooks aloud to him.

We learned in Reversals that parents need to help their child discover his gifts, outside the academic realm. When his self-esteem is under assault every day at school, he needs to find a place where he feels smart, skillful, successful. It could be art or tennis, theater or baseball, dance or model airplanes. For Jon, it was music. He played the string bass. Looking back, Jon says he didn't have any trouble learning to read music. "That's because it's not words," he observes. "It's pictures."

In the meantime, I had started to educate myself on special education—the science, the terminology, the law—and the then-current strategies for teaching kids with learning disabilities. Before I knew what was happening, I was an activist. From the school district's special-ed parent advisory council, I went on to state-level work on various councils and committees, including a stint as a governor's appointee to the Oregon Advisory Council to Special Education. A two-year term as president of the Oregon Branch of the International Dyslexia Association gave me the chance to work with professionals and advocates all over the country. The experience reminded me with fresh force about the urgent need for action on behalf of the nation's 10 million dyslexic students and the many million more who may not have a biological glitch, but whose reading has been hobbled by inadequate instruction.

As for Jon, the little boy who couldn't read graduated from the University of Oregon in 2004 with a 3.2 GPA in his double majors, Spanish and international studies. He also completed minors in Latin American studies and international business. He spent his junior year studying in Cuernavaca, Mexico, where he polished up his Spanish. As I write this, Jon has joined the Peace Corps and is getting ready for a two-year stint in Latin America. "If you see my ninth-grade Spanish teacher," he said, "tell her what I'm doing." Living well, it seems, is Jon's best revenge for the teacher who tried to oust him from her class when he hit a wall on written grammar and verb conjugations.

Still, Jon's face reveals some residual sadness when he talks about being a little kid. "My first memory of school was being in kindergarten and trying to write my name, and not really being able to do that," he says. "It's not a good feeling, not being able to write your name." As he moved through the early grades, things only got worse. Elementary school, he says, "made me cry." He remembers his teachers telling him he "just needed to work harder."

"Third grade kind of sticks out to me as a hard year just because everyone could read and I couldn't," he says. "People were reading stories like *James and the Giant Peach*, and I couldn't. And SSR [silent sustained reading] was just the worst time in my life, because there's nothing to do if you can't read. You just sit there, twenty minutes of pretending to read. All I could do was look at the words—I had no concept of what they meant. It was *excruciating*."

On the day of Jon's college graduation, whenever I snuck a motherly glance in his direction, I found myself thinking about what it had taken to get him to that moment—to the celebratory hoist of a beer in the very kitchen where I once hovered as a young mom, anxiously eavesdropping on his tutoring sessions. The dining room table—now piled with chips and salsa and the wild Pacific salmon that Jon's dad had smoked in the garage for the occasion—was the same table where Jon had sat with his tutor on all those afternoons, all those years ago, in his agonizing journey to become a reader. As I watched my son, so confident about his future, a little shiver passed over me. What if Jon *hadn't* gotten the help he got? What if?

A COCKTAIL OF DISABILITIES

In recent years, a lot of old theories about learning disabilities have been discredited. Among the ideas that science has trashed:

- That learning disabled kids see backwards or upside-down and hence are more likely to reverse letters and numbers (not so, researchers now say).
- That boys are more likely to be LD (girls just don't get identified as often because they tend to behave nicely in school).
- That learning disabilities stem from poor parenting or laziness (not a whiff of truth).
- That LD kids will "grow out of it" (in fact, learning disabilities are life-long conditions).

"The greatest stumbling block preventing a dyslexic child from realizing his potential and following his dreams," writes Yale University researcher Sally Shaywitz in her 2003 book *Overcoming Dyslexia*, "is the widespread ignorance about the true nature of dyslexia" (89).

Despite the diligence of researchers who have been chipping away at the myths ever since learning disabilities were officially recognized by the federal government in the late 1960s, many misconceptions have hung on stubbornly. But a couple of scientific advances that coincided in the mid-1990s are quietly revolutionizing the field. Powerful new technologies have let research teams at the University of Washington and Yale capture real-time images of the brain at work. And the monumental Human Genome Project, which mapped the infinitely complex genetic code, has helped unmask other clues for these and other teams funded by the National Institute of Child Health and Human Development (NICHD)—one of twenty-seven institutes and centers comprising the National Institutes of Health.

Learning disabilities, it turns out, stem from faulty wiring in the brain— what Shaywitz calls a "glitch" (2003, 17) that forms in early stages of embryonic development. "This miswiring," she says, "is confined to a specific neural system" (17) used for reading. LD kids—far from slacking off— are working mightily when they tackle even the simplest language tasks. In fact, in a 1999 test involving word pairs, they used nearly five times the brain area as other kids, the UW team found. The brain imaging tools reveal a clear "neural signature"—that is, a distinct pattern of brain activity for disabled readers. "If you have a broken arm, we can see that on an x-ray," Shaywitz told *Education Week*. "These brain-activated patterns now provide evidence for what has previously been a hidden disability" (Manzo 1998, 7).

The other big new finding: Learning disabilities have a genetic link. Just as kids can inherit olive skin, migraines, or musical talent from Grandma, so, too, can they inherit her learning disorder. Of the twenty genes associated with the reading process, UW researchers Jennifer Thomson and Wendy Raskind recently singled out several possible sites on five different chromosomes that have been implicated in reading and writing disorders. These discoveries constitute a death blow to the widely held notion that learning disabilities don't really exist—that kids with normal intelligence who struggle to learn just aren't trying hard enough or aren't getting enough support from Mom and Dad. Shaywitz, offering encouragement to the parents of disabled readers, said, "You will not accept allusions to a temporary or developmental lag or that 'some children are just slow readers' or that girls are not dyslexic. Nor will you accept that there is 'no such thing as dyslexia.' Anyone who says this needs to be educated" (2003, 129).

As knowledge about learning disabilities has grown, so have the numbers. Fewer than 800,000 kids were identified as LD in the mid-1970s. But by the middle of the 1990s, that figure had swelled to 2.5 million, according to the U.S. Department of Education. By the new millennium, LD kids accounted for half of all placements into special ed.

The ways kids can be disabled vary. In her classic textbook *Learning Disabilities: Theories, Diagnosis, and Teaching Strategies*, Janet Lerner, a professor of education at Northeastern Illinois University, identifies several types of learning disabilities. She defines dyslexia as "a severe reading disorder in which the individual cannot learn to read or does not acquire fluent and efficient reading skills" (2003, G-3). Other learning disabilities include dysgraphia ("extremely poor handwriting or the inability to perform the motor movements required for handwriting" (G-3) and dyscalculia ("a medical term indicating lack of ability to perform mathematical functions") (G-3). Each of these conditions, she says, is associated with "neurological dysfunction" (2003, G-3).

Lerner then goes on to describe several related problem areas that tend to show up in the same kids: auditory discrimination ("the ability to recognize a difference between phoneme sounds; also the ability to identify words that are the same and words that are different when the difference is a single phoneme element, for example, *big-pig*") (G-1), visual discrimination ("the ability to note visual differences or similarities between objects, including letters and words") (G-9), and attention deficit disorder/attention deficit hyperactivity disorder (ADD/ADHD) ("difficulty in concentrating and staying on a task," with or without hyperactivity) (G-1).

Although learning disabilities have distinct names, they typically occur in clusters rather than in isolation. People who have trouble reading, for instance, very often have trouble writing, too. Other problems, such as attention deficit disorder, complicate the picture even further. For example, 30 percent of people with learning disabilities also struggle with attention disorders. "Disabilities don't fit into neat categories," Pat Wingert and Barbara Kantrowitz explain in a 1997 *Newsweek* piece. "They are more likely to be a cocktail of disability types and associated problems" (56).

BRAIN WAVES

Of the various disorders, dyslexia is by far the most common (hence, the most widely studied and well understood). Estimates of dyslexia among students range from 5 percent to 20 percent, nationwide. The University of Washington, in a 2000 press release, puts the proportion of dyslexic kids at between 5 percent and 15 percent of all students. Shaywitz, who conducted a long-term study of 450 Connecticut kids beginning in 1983, categorized 20 percent of the children as reading disabled. That's one in five kids, adding up to at least 10 million children across the United States.

But a "reading disability" does not necessarily mean dyslexia. Lyon contends that among the typical 20 percent of troubled readers (those who have "substantial difficulties" learning to read), only half or fewer are truly dyslexic. Rather, reading disability falls along a continuum. "There is no natural joint separating dyslexic and good readers," Shaywitz explains (2003, 28). Nor is there a line dividing dyslexic children from kids whose reading struggles originate in other causes. Citing the Connecticut study, as well as findings from Britain and New Zealand, she describes reading ability and reading disability as "an unbroken continuum" (28).

Where each child falls on that continuum depends on a unique blend of genes, environment, and what Thomson and Raskind call "stochastic processes"—what most of us term "chance events." And that's where a gray mist rolls in to cloud the landscape of diagnosis and treatment. With this "disability," hidden behind the façade of a smart child who is very often clever and creative, the designation of "LD" can be tough to make. And what about normal-IQ kids who struggle to read, yet don't have that telltale "neural signature"? Sorting out the infinite gradations of learning difficulties can boggle the best of teachers.

Lyon and others argue that countless kids are being mistakenly labeled as disabled—that with the right instruction at the right time, these at-risk students would be spared the trauma of special-ed placement and all the emotional baggage it carries. Unnecessary special services can be a costly drain in this era of budgets worn thin by tax revolts, slumping markets, and rising energy prices—an era when many schools are hard-pressed to fund separate programs for lagging learners. The lion's share of kids who, to use Lyon's words, "hit the wall" in reading are not actually disabled but are instead NBT—"never been taught." Timely teaching with scientifically supported strategies can negate the need for pricey intervention for all but the most disabled.

"Researchers suspect there's a window between the ages of five and seven when the underlying skills of reading are most easily learned," Kantrowitz and Anne Underwood wrote in a November 1999 *Newsweek* article (72). They note that a kindergarten teacher can accomplish in thirty minutes what a fourth-grade teacher would need two hours to do. Extrapolate those figures to the sixth or seventh grades—the time when many LD kids finally start getting help—and you begin to get a sense of the costs of waiting.

Read the research literature about what kind of intervention LD kids need, and you'll find two words turning up again and again: "early" and "appropriate." No one really argues about what "early" means. As noted above, the jury is in on third grade as the pivot point for long-term reading proficiency. But when you take up the topic of what's "appropriate," you'd better put on a heat shield. That's because you've dropped a match into the most explosive cauldron of educational philosophy: whole language versus phonics.

The ancient debate about direct instruction versus discovery learning crystallizes clearly in the field of reading disabilities. Here's why: A mounting body of evidence shows that struggling readers—both the truly disabled as well as the chronically confused—lack a skill that is absolutely essential to the reading process: phonemic awareness. Simply put, it's the ability to hear the individual sounds in spoken words. The typical disabled reader can't distinguish those sounds (called phonemes), so she fails to make the next leap—linking sounds to letters. Without these basic building blocks, the rest of the reading skills—decoding, word recognition, and reading comprehension—are all but impossible.

Researchers point to this deficit as a critical clue to the riddle of dyslexia, the puzzling phenomenon of children who, to use the language of Lyon, have "average or above average intelligence, robust oral language experience, and frequent interactions with books" yet are stumped by print (1996b, R18). He notes that many of the children studied under the National Institutes of Health-funded research have been read to regularly since infancy, have well-developed speaking vocabularies, and "can quickly understand and discuss in rich detail" the content of text read aloud to them. Yet they "flounder" when they try to read age-appropriate material on their own (R18).

The nub of the problem lies in whether kids can grasp the "alphabetic principle" on which the English language rests. To read the language, Lyon explains in the *Washington Post*, one must "unlock the relationships" between forty sounds and twenty-six letters. Research has taught us, he says, that "in order for a beginning reader to learn how to map or translate printed symbols (letters and letter patterns) to sound, he or she must intuitively understand that speech can be segmented, and that segmented units of speech can be represented by printed forms"—an awareness that to most of us seems "so easy and commonplace that we take it for granted" (1996b, R18). But recent findings in university laboratories have turned up a juicy tidbit: It is not the ear that helps children understand that a spoken word like "cat" is divided into three sounds and that these sounds can be mapped onto the letters /c/, /a/, and /t/. Rather, it is the brain. "In many individuals," Lyon says, "the brain is not processing this type of linguistic phonological information in an efficient manner" (R18).

A Yale study published in the journal *Biological Psychiatry* on July 15, 2002, found that dyslexia is linked to a particular region of the brain, which shows disruptions in affected children. The researchers found that dyslexic children compensate by learning to read with other parts of their brain. "Dyslexic children can't use the highly specialized area [of the brain] that is activated in good readers and therefore don't read automatically or fluently," lead author Bennett Shaywitz told *Education Daily* in July 2002. "Because they develop compensatory systems on the front and right side of the brain, they read more accurately over time, but remain slow readers" (Rubin, 2002).

Based on these and other findings—including the 2000 report of the National Reading Panel—Lyon and colleagues argue convincingly for early reading instruction that's rich in lessons about the sound–letter relationship. "Disabled readers must be presented highly structured, explicit, and intensive instruction in phonics rules and the application of the rules to print," he says. "Longitudinal data indicate that systematic, structured phonics instruction results in more favorable outcomes in reading than does a context emphasis" (1996a).

Contrary to the old-style "drill-and-kill" approach to phonics in which kids sat at their desks, dazed by mind-numbing flash cards and other rote exercises, instruction in the sound–letter link can be developmentally appropriate—even fun. Researcher Virginia Berninger, a principal investigator for the multidisciplinary Learning Disabilities Center at the University of Washington, has developed a package of materials with the Psychological Corporation called PAL (Process Assessment of the Learner). Published in 1998 by Harcourt Brace, the *PAL Guides for Intervention: Reading and Writing* offers a collection of research-based "sound games" and "looking games" for first-

and second-graders that take only about ten minutes and boost kids' word skills significantly.

Researchers are in agreement, though, that a curriculum that is all phonics and no context ("real reading in real books") is a loser. Just as the National Research Council stressed in its important 1998 report *Preventing Reading Difficulties in Young Children*, "balance" is the place to be. Notes Lyon,

> A number of National Institutes of Health studies being conducted at different research sites have all reported that a balanced instructional program composed of direct instruction in phonological awareness, phonics, and contextual reading is necessary for gains in reading skills to be achieved. Without a doubt, we have found that teaching methods that are based upon only one philosophy, such as "the whole-language approach" or "the phonics method," are counterproductive for children with reading disabilities. No matter how bright the child and how interesting the reading material, a child will not learn to read unless he or she understands how print is translated into sound. Likewise, no matter how much phonological awareness and phonics knowledge a youngster has, the child will not want to engage in reading and writing unless it is meaningful and interesting and taught in an exciting and vibrant fashion. (1996b, R18)

The brain glitch in the neurological reading pathways of dyslexic kids *should* be only that—a "minor malfunction or snag"—in their educational careers, because science and experience have shown us that they *can* be taught to read and go on to succeed in school and in life. The teaching methods that foster this success have been available for decades. But there's a bigger glitch in the way. If the glitch in the brain wiring of dyslexic kids is a "micro-glitch," the instructional glitch in U.S. public schools is a "macro-glitch." This systemic glitch—the widespread misconceptions about reading acquisition and dyslexia, the lukewarm belief that *all* children really *can* learn to read, and the wholesale reliance on uninformed instruction—compounds the malfunction of individual brain wiring by an order of magnitude of millions. It not only inflicts lifelong disability and emotional devastation on dyslexic kids but it also undercuts the life chances of countless other children who fall elsewhere along the continuum of reading troubles.

Seeing the statistics in black and white should feel like a sucker punch to anyone who cares about kids. Nearly 40 percent of America's fourth-graders are unable to read at a fourth-grade level, according to the 2001 "nation's report card" of the National Center for Education Statistics. Forty percent: an astounding figure for the most prosperous nation and the greatest democracy on earth. "The bottom line," Lyon said in a 2004 interview with David Boulton, coproducer and creator of an education and public awareness project called Children of the Code, "is for a country like America to be leaving behind . . . 40 percent of its youngsters in terms of not being able to read is unconscionable."

2

The Reading Wars: Four Hundred Years of Stalemate

It is mysterious how these educational theories came to be associated so mindlessly with politics.

—E. D. Hirsch, Jr., *Educational Leadership*, 2001

How we teach our children shifts with the winds of philosophies and politics, leaving many observers dizzy and dismayed.

—Alan B. Krueger, Princeton University, 1999

Mankind likes to think in terms of extreme opposites. It is given to formulating its beliefs in terms of Either-Ors, between which it recognizes no intermediate possibilities. . . . Educational philosophy is no exception.

—John Dewey, *Experience and Education*, 1939

Reid Lyon, his shock of prematurely white hair clearly visible from the farthest corners of the cavernous conference room, was speaking with the intensity of a guy who has too much to say for the hour allotted. As he stood at the podium, describing his team's "cradle-to-grave" research on how people learn to read, a piercing, high-pitched squeal suddenly shrieked from the microphone. Some of his listeners winced and covered their ears until a technician rushed up and fiddled with the mike. When Lyon resumed, he cracked, "I thought it was something Ken Goodman was doing."

It was an inside joke—one that got an appreciative snicker from many of those in attendance at the 2003 annual conference of the International Dyslexia Association. Kenneth S. Goodman, the widely acknowledged "father of whole language," is Reid Lyon's nemesis in the struggle for the hearts and

minds of American teachers. As Lyon and the team of researchers he led for
the National Institutes of Health during the 1990s and early 2000s gradually
undercut the dominance of whole language in the long-standing fight over
how kids learn to read, Goodman has fought back with regular counter-
punches. "Kenneth Goodman is not known for his silence," journalist Kath-
leen Kennedy Manzo wrote in *Education Week* on March 3, 2004. "The
professor emeritus at the University of Arizona," she explained, "has been
wont to interrupt conference sessions or speak bluntly at public hearings to
deride what he sees as lockstep, skills-based approaches to instruction or narrow views of reading research" (11).

In that particular instance, Manzo was reporting on Goodman's call for
a boycott of the May 2004 annual convention of the International Reading
Association, where Lyon was on the roster as a keynote speaker. Goodman,
posting his objections on a listserv for reading teachers and scholars, accused
Lyon of helping to establish "a narrow and exclusive definition of reading
research in federal and state laws and marginalizing and blacklisting
researchers, research methodologies, and research paradigms" (Manzo 2004,
11). Those being marginalized, presumably, are Goodman and his ilk. A few
months later, during a live "Web chat" sponsored by *Ed Week* featuring Lyon,
an irate message from Goodman popped up online. "I deeply resent," Goodman huffed during the October 28 discussion, "your characterizing the view
of Reid Lyon as THE [*sic*] scientific approach to reading instruction and
development."

Goodman has gone so far as to compare himself to such exalted thinkers
from history as Galileo and Copernicus, the Renaissance astronomers who
were persecuted for challenging the earth's central position in the universe.
In a letter to the editor published in *Ed Week* on February 13, 2002, Goodman
called the current federal support for Lyon's brand of reading research an
"inquisition" that brands other points of view as "heretical" (48).

David Ziffer of *I Can Read!* fired back with both barrels, countering in *his*
letter to *Ed Week* on February 27, 2002, that Goodman's comparing himself
to Galileo gets the facts exactly backwards. As Ziffer explained,

> In the time of Galileo, [it was] the authorities [who] were steeped in misguided
> superstition, subscribing to scientifically unsupported doctrine. . . . Today, it is the
> authorities [i.e., the U.S. Department of Education, the National Institutes of Health,
> university researchers] who are looking to science, and Mr. Goodman and his col-
> leagues who seem to be looking to the black arts for guidance in the subject of read-
> ing instruction. (40)

A further lob into the *Ed Week* editorial volley came from Lisa Leppin of The
Classical Tutor in Wisconsin, who reproached Goodman for peddling meth-

ods "that have been less adequately tested than hairspray and bubblegum" (40).

Charges of dark-side motives are not out of the ordinary among the reading warriors. Adherents to both perspectives have, over the years, flung around some rather startling accusations. The most over-the-top dialogue seems to borrow imagery from the gothic tales of Transylvania and from the hell-and-damnation ranting of revivalist preachers, leading tents full of sinners to repentance. The moralistic tenor of the debate is a perfect echo of the larger culture wars raging all over America in city halls and state legislatures, in churches, temples, and synagogues, on talk radio and editorial pages. As improbable as it seems, reading instruction has gotten tangled up in the ideological debate over the "three *g*'s"—God, guns, and gays—to borrow a radio talk-show catch-phrase for the culture wars.

At the 1997 meeting of the Society for the Scientific Study of Reading (SSSR), one leading researcher told several hair-curling horror stories from her personal experience. The events recounted by Linnea C. Ehri of the City University of New York Graduate School convey the down-and-dirty tone of the dispute. She told her colleagues,

> I recall attending a symposium entitled "Researching Whole Language" at the 1989 AERA [American Educational Research Association] meeting. [Fellow researchers] Rich West, Keith Stanovich, and I stood at the back of a very crowded room. We found ourselves the target of criticism as one speaker contrasted whole-language research with traditional research. . . . He branded these [traditional] researchers as "academic rapists." This was clearly an attitude-shaping tactic intended to turn educators against an approach to research that had produced evidence challenging whole-language beliefs. (1998, 111)

A second anecdote from Ehri, who was then president of the SSSR, adds further illustration:

> Another example of the use of maligning language to prejudice educators occurred during a conference that was organized by IRA and the Center for the Study of Reading for the purpose of presenting the latest research to publishers of reading programs. Marilyn Adams was on the program talking about the book she had just written, *Beginning to Read: Thinking and Learning about Print*, which reviewed much of the research on beginning reading processes that I and others had published. Joanna Williams [of Teachers College of Columbia University] and I were discussants for Marilyn's presentation. Later in the day, another discussant who was a whole-language advocate expressed disagreement with Adams and branded all of us "phonicators." [Read more about the phonicators later in this chapter.] Since then, Marilyn has been the target of many such attacks. Her book has been referred to as the work of the devil. At an IRA meeting, many people heard a whole-language

leader assert publicly that Marilyn should be "shot with a silver bullet," implying that she was a vampire. (1998, 112)

(In European folklore, it was actually the werewolf who was vulnerable to the silver bullet, while the vampire was cut down by a stake in the heart.)

At the same meeting, Ehri also related a run-in she had with Ken Goodman early in her career. She had written a paper that suggested how Goodman's theory of reading acquisition "could be elaborated to explain more completely how word recognition works as readers' eyes move across a page and get meaning from print." She sent off a copy to the professor for feedback. "He returned it with his comments in the margins," Ehri said. "These consisted mainly of the word 'No' repeated two or three times on every page, sometimes underlined. His final comment at the end consisted of a sentence declaring that reading is not a process of identifying words." She was stunned. "I was unprepared," she confessed, "for a reaction so closed-minded and dogmatic" (1998, 100).

DÉJÀ VU ALL OVER AGAIN

The feud between Reid Lyon and Ken Goodman is only the current personification of a debate that has raged, literally, for centuries. Although these two prominent figures embody the two main camps of today's reading wars, their predecessors in this epic intellectual contest go back four hundred years. Pioneering Harvard reading researcher Jean Chall, in her now-classic 1967 work *Learning to Read: The Great Debate* (commonly referred to simply as *The Great Debate*), observes, "Our age is not the first to produce 'new' approaches to beginning reading instruction" (13). She cites the 1962 book *Linguistics and Reading* by Charles C. Fries, which reviews "courses of study, manuals, and journal articles published between 1570 and 1900 [that] uncovers a succession of 'discoveries' and 'rediscoveries'—alphabet reforms, word methods, sentence methods, experience methods, phonic methods—each with its claim to be the 'new,' the 'natural,' 'true,' 'logical,' way to begin. By ignoring the dates of publication, we can easily believe we are reading current reports" (Chall 1967, 13).

Almost forty years after Chall's observation, having turned the corner on yet another century—indeed, on another millennium—we can *still* believe we are reading current reports in those centuries-old papers. You can almost see Chall shaking her head as she asks, rhetorically, in the 1983 update of *The Great Debate,* "How is it possible that during a time of growing research evidence, some of the statements on various issues of the debate seem as heated as in 1967—and in 1841?" (44).

Fries drives home the stubbornness of the reading controversy in his book, which he describes as "a survey of past practice and theory in the teaching of reading." Declaring that "the discussions in English concerning the methods and materials for the teaching of reading began at least four hundred years ago" (1962, 1), Fries, like Chall, points out that in the reading wars, "new" theories are actually retrofitted ideas from decades past. "The chief methods and combinations of methods now discussed so vigorously were actually in use long before the time of modern educational research," the University of Michigan professor writes (6). Theories of reading come and go like clothing trends—like girls in 2005 sporting the "new" hip-hugger bell-bottoms that their grandmothers wore to Joan Baez concerts in the 1960s; like the cycles of hemlines, from mini to maxi to midi and back again; like the ups and downs of heels, from spikes to Earth shoes to platforms to Birkenstocks—from pretty to practical, sexy to sensible.

While science marches forward in every other field, reading instruction spins in the repetitive cycles of fashion and fad. As Rudolph Flesch observed in the sequel to his 1955 bestseller, *Why Johnny Can't Read*, Goodman, along with his wife, Yetta Goodman, and another psycholinguist named Frank Smith, "invented a new science to clothe shabby old look-and-say in shiny new garments" (1981, 23–24).

Fries's historical chronology begins with a discussion of a sixteenth-century book by an Englishman named John Hart, a critic of the then-favored "alphabetic method," in which students would spell a word by naming the letters and then pronounce it. Hart's little book, published in 1570, bore the weighty title *A Methode or comfortable beginning for all unlearned, whereby they may bee taught to read English, in a very short time, with pleasure* (Edward de Vere Newsletter 2001, 1). Hart proposed revamping the alphabet to make it more phonetic as an aid to young readers.

Hart's ponderous title, with its archaic spelling and syntax, seems quaint today. English language usage has marched on, and modern book editors, who favor pithy titles, would be scandalized by the on-and-on moniker. Even more scandalous, though, is the realization that the debate has barely budged since Hart's book made its debut during the Renaissance and the Protestant Reformation—that educators are still quarreling about ideas that were being argued in the days of bloodletting by lance and by leech. When Hart wrote his little book, William Shakespeare's first plays—Henry VI, Parts I, II, and II—were still twenty years from hitting the stage. Just seven years before, bubonic plague had swept across Europe, wiping out 20,000 in London alone.

And it would be another fifty years before the Pilgrims would set sail for Plymouth.

In the centuries since Hart wrote his book, science has brought us not only automobiles but hydrogen-powered engines. It has given us not only the discovery of germs, but antibiotics to fight them. Not only telescopes, but color photos shot by a robot roving over the surface of Mars. Not only an understanding of mental illnesses, but antidepressants, psychotropic drugs, and psychotherapy to treat them.

Science has also given us a real-time look at the disparate brain activity of struggling readers. And it has demonstrated over and over the superior effectiveness of direct instruction in phonics over a meaning-based approach for beginning reading. Yet countless educators continue to hang on to theories that are the educational equivalent of a green-cheese moon, or demon-induced dementia.

Education's Uncivil War

The debate, spilling first from the pens of thinkers across the Atlantic scrawling alone in their quarters on quiet campuses, has gathered its momentum and venom through a revolution in personal writing technologies—from goose quills and steel nibs through fountain pens and ballpoints, to clunky manual Underwoods and streamlined Selectric typewriters, all the way to supercompact notebook computers propped on jetliner tray tables at 30,000 feet.

By the time the twentieth century had reached its midpoint, reading methods were being debated not only among scholars and classroom teachers but also among ordinary citizens. The debate had by then crossed the pond and was raging in the United States, Australia, and New Zealand. Parents took sides, politicians weighed in.

By the 1950s, the tone of the quarrel was at a full, rolling boil. Flesch's 1955 blockbuster book lashed out angrily at what in those days was called the "look, say" (or "look-and-say") method. By the 1980s, fed by countless articles in both the academic and popular presses, the debate had erupted into a bona fide pedagogical conflagration. Despite current calls for consensus, for "balance," for a cool appraisal of the facts, the fight smolders on.

Writers trying to be circumspect have referred to the reading controversy as the "great debate" or the "reading crisis." The more common term is "the reading wars," less genteel but more to the point. Portraying the clash in militaristic terms better captures the ferocity of what is really more like trench warfare than trenchant discussion. From its roots in philosophy, linguistics, epistemology, pedagogy, and psychology, the debate has degenerated into a bitter, partisan battle—more Hatfield-and-McCoy feud than Socratic dialogue.

Tragically for millions of students, the invective and side-taking have impeded reason and blocked progress in a branch of learning that, quite literally, determines success or failure for schoolchildren. Even as experts across the nation call for a truce, there are thousands of whole-language diehards who have no intention of waving the white flag. The collateral damage in this fight-to-the-death battle is kids, particularly kids from disadvantaged backgrounds and kids with dyslexia. Military leaders will tell you that in any war, there are "acceptable losses" for whatever greater good is gained. Ironically, that greater good—the well-being of children—is the very thing that is being sacrificed as the two sides duke it out.

Out of Whole Cloth

One of the early thinkers who laid the philosophical groundwork for today's bankrupt reading policies was an eighteenth-century professor from Berlin named Friedrich Gedike. In 1791, Gedike described reading as a sort of mystical process of conjecture in a book titled *Children's Book for the First Practice in Reading without the ABC's and Spelling*, which Flesch credits with being the original look-and-say primer (1981, 16). In the preface to this primer, Gedike explained his theory: "Through the mysterious sense of analogy [the child] will increasingly find out words on his own or, if you will, learn to guess. At the same time, he will sense, even more mysteriously, why it must be this word and no other" (Flesch 1981, 16).

Two hundred years later, Goodman dredged up Gedike's notion and launched the modern whole-language movement when he famously described reading as a "psycholinguistic guessing game." Because language is predictable—that is, it conforms to certain structural rules—readers can nimbly guess their way through written text, explain Goodman disciples Carole Edelsky, Bess Altwerger, and Barbara Flores in their 1991 book *Whole Language: What's the Difference?*

Goodman's theory was embraced by the education community, which was already primed. Beginning in about 1930, teachers had formed a near-unanimous consensus in favor of meaning-emphasis approaches, according to Chall. By the late 1930s, the "Dick and Jane" series had taken the nation by storm with its "word method" or "look-and-say" approach. Although the Scott, Foresman and Co. series was not whole language as a purist would define it today, it was a precursor in that it taught students to learn words as meaningful "wholes," rather than breaking them down into their letter and sound components. Chall surveyed reading-methods textbooks and found that between 1955 and 1965, more than 80 percent recommended a meaning emphasis, with the rest favoring a combined approach. Not a single textbook recommended a code emphasis during that decade.

Even then, the word method was not a new notion. The idea had been around since at least the early 1800s, hinging on the belief that kids should learn whole words first because words are "meaning units"—that is, they denote a thing or a place or a person or an action, something that holds meaning for the beginning reader. Letters and syllables, in contrast, are abstractions devoid of intrinsic meaning. Significantly, these early word-method programs did not shun phonics instruction. Rather, they introduced phonetics after the child had learned a certain number of words by sight or had finished several lessons.

The hegemony of meaning-based programs during this period was not, however, absolute, at least among scholars. The field of linguistics—the scientific study of the nature of language—was grappling with the reading process along with the fields of psychology, philosophy, and education. As early as 1942, there were linguists who argued that the major task in beginning reading is learning to recognize words in their printed form—to decipher the written symbols that stand for the spoken words that stand for the objects and ideas that are familiar to little kids. A kindergartner already *knows* the meaning of the word "cat." The thing he *doesn't* know is that those three marks, the letters /c/, /a/, and /t/, are the written representation of that well-known word, the one that refers to the next-door neighbor's fat, tail-flicking tabby. "The first-grader, the linguists felt, already knows the meanings of the words he reads; therefore, meaning is really not the instructional problem," Chall said (1967, 66).

One of the most distinguished of those linguistic scholars, Leonard Bloomfield, criticized the then-prevailing approach to beginning reading. "Since the child comes to school with a considerable command of spoken language, he reasoned, reading instruction should begin by teaching him the printed equivalents for his oral vocabulary," Chall said. "Meaning, considered so important by authors of conventional programs, comes naturally as the code is broken, Bloomfield argued, since the words in the first readers are already part of the child's listening and speaking vocabulary" (1967, 29).

Despite the arguments of Bloomfield and others, holistic reading instruction prevailed until the mid-1970s. Then, largely under the influence of Chall's landmark study, textbooks for teachers shifted from a mostly meaning-emphasis to some preference for a combined, eclectic approach (38 percent). The other two-thirds were split between those favoring a meaning emphasis and those favoring a code emphasis (Chall 1983). The Public Broadcasting Service children's television shows Sesame Street and Electric

Company appeared, giving new life to phonics by teaching letters and sounds directly in a fun format. Despite these nods to Chall's pro-phonics findings, however, the impact on actual classroom practice appears to have been negligible. In *Why Johnny Still Can't Read: A New Look at the Scandal of Our Schools*—the 1981 sequel to his earlier treatise—Flesch saw barely a budge:

> There are two schools of thought about how to teach a child to read. One is called "intensive phonics" or "systematic phonics" or, more recently, "decoding" or "code emphasis." . . . I'll call it "phonics-first." The other is called the "look-and-say" or "whole-word" or "sight-reading" method or—so help me—"psycholinguistics." I'll use "look-and-say." When I wrote my book *Why Johnny Can't Read* twenty-five years ago, look-and-say ruled supreme. Almost all American schools used it. Phonics-first was a poor orphan, used only in a handful of schools. I said in my book that phonics-first worked splendidly and should be used in all schools, while look-and-say was wretchedly poor and should be abandoned at once. Unfortunately, my advice fell on deaf ears. With heart-breaking slowness, phonics-first crept into some 15 percent of our schools, but an estimated 85 percent of them still stick to old, discredited look-and-say. The results of this mass miseducation have been disastrous. (1)

Even as millions of American children were undergoing the saccharine antics of Dick, Jane, Spot, Sally, and Puff, look-and-say was morphing into the modern whole-language movement. Appropriating and expanding on the ideas of earlier holistic theorists, the new holism argued that learning to read is no different from learning to speak and that lessons on letters and sounds are not "natural." As Gedike had posited, "real reading" is separate from discrete skills—it is a transcendent, almost supernatural experience, not tethered to niggling details like letters and sounds.

But the "new" meaning-emphasis theories promoted by Goodman and others were considerably more radical than those of earlier thinkers. Staking out a position far more extreme than earlier meaning-based approaches, the new holists not only marginalized skills, they ran them out of town on a rail. Citing the 1977 writings of San Diego State University education professor Patrick Groff, Chall notes that whole language as envisioned by Goodman and his followers is based solely on a "sight approach to reading, with *no teaching of phonics, not even 'later and less' phonics* combined with context and picture clues characteristic of the meaning-emphasis programs common from the 1920s to 1950s" (1983, 38, italics added).

Regie Routman, the beloved whole-language author of such hugely successful books for teachers as *Transitions*, published in 1988, and *Invitations*, published in 1994, has gone so far as to dismiss the utility of vowels. "Routman's activities," notes Adams, "are focused on initial and final consonants:

The vowels, she submits, are generally unnecessary for printed word recognition" (1998, 84).

This notion's preposterousness can be demonstrated with one quick example. Think of the meanings of the following two sentences—sentences that differ by two little vowels: "The blond man reached under the counter and took out the gun" versus "The blind man reached under the counter and took out the gin."

In Pursuit of Progress

Cathy Wyrick rummages through her tote bag excitedly. "I want to show you a couple of things," says the cofounder and director of the Blosser Center for Dyslexia Resources in Portland, Oregon. Her tone, as she tenderly, gingerly lays three or four scuffed and faded little books on the table, is almost reverent. "These," she tells us, "are antiques." With the flushed pride of a collector who has snagged a coveted treasure, Wyrick displays her relics of American education: a *Webster's Speller* from 1810, the *McGuffey's Readers*, ubiquitous in U.S. schools in the nineteenth century, and *Appleton's School Readers*, another popular nineteenth-century series.

Wyrick's improbable fondness for these homely little volumes grew from a deeply personal quest: to figure out how we, as a nation, got to this impasse in reading instruction. Why, she wondered as she watched her dyslexic daughter struggle in school, did educators reject a systematic, code-based approach to teaching kids to read? What were the intellectual roots of whole language?

And so she became a familiar presence in Portland's libraries and bookstores, scouring their collections on philosophy, neurology, psychology, and education for clues. She wanted to know, How did an argument over skills versus meaning in reading instruction endure for centuries to become fodder for pundit, press, parent, politician, and even pulpit? How did phonics become a shibboleth of conservatism, and whole language the salvation of liberalism? How did reading instruction take its place with abortion, school prayer, gun control, and, most recently, stem-cell research and gay marriage, in the "culture wars" that have divided America right down the middle at this tender edge of the third millennium?

What Wyrick found was a division that cuts much deeper than mere methods. The reading wars, she discovered, go to the very core of the perceived purposes of public education. Calling for more democratic schooling, progressive scholars at the turn of the twentieth century fueled the movement away from such phonics-heavy mainstays as Ginn and Company's Beacon

Readers, which they viewed as top-down, authoritarian, and antithetical to free and independent thinking.

But in a controversy that is riddled with ironies, this laudable gesture for democratic ideals has backfired. The unintended consequence of abandoning phonics has been a greater rift between rich and poor. The kids who most desperately need instruction in the alphabetic code—those from disadvantaged homes where books and newspapers and magazines are rare or absent—are cut out of the literacy loop when schools withhold the key to reading that, for most middle-class kids, is a birthright.

Recent data show a yawning gap between rich and poor. In 2003, 55 percent of fourth-graders who were eligible for free or reduced-price lunch scored below "basic" reading level on the "nation's report card" (the National Assessment of Educational Progress). Only 24 percent of the other kids fell into that bottom slot. Looking at the numbers another way, only 45 percent of poor fourth-graders were at or above basic, while 76 percent of the more affluent students reached the basic level or higher. A mere 15 percent of poor children were proficient readers, but 42 percent of wealthier children reached that upper rung (National Center for Education Statistics, 2003b).

Arguably, the two most prominent early twentieth-century thinkers responsible for launching the theories that revolutionized education in the United States were John Dewey and Jean Piaget. Dewey, an American philosopher, and Piaget, a Swiss psychologist, were among the originators of the theory of "constructivism"—that is, learners create their own understandings by blending new information and ideas with what they already know. The practices that educators today call "child-centered"—active learning, discovery learning, developmentally appropriate practices—all grew out of this school of thought, which can, in turn, be traced to Enlightenment philosopher Jean-Jacques Rousseau, who said, "Give your pupil no lesson in words, he must learn from his experience" (Weir 1990).

One author of the reemerging holistic or meaning-based theory of reading instruction was a psychology professor at Clark University named Edmund Burke Huey. Repackaging the notions put forth by Gedike a century before, Huey's 1908 treatise, *The Psychology and Pedagogy of Reading* (reprinted in 1968), put a new spin on the old ideas. "It instantly became the bible of the movement," Flesch said (1981, 21). Huey made this declaration:

If [a child] grasps, approximately, the total meaning of the sentence in which (a) new word stands, he has read the sentence. . . . And even if the child substitutes words of his own for some that are on the page, provided that these express the meaning, it is an encouraging sign that the reading has been real, and recognition of details will come as it is needed. The shock that such a statement will give to many a practical teacher of reading is but an accurate measure of the hold that a false ideal has taken of us, viz, that to read is to say just what is upon the page, instead of to think, each in his own way, the meaning the page suggests. (Huey 1968, 349)

Fast-forward yet another century, and Huey's theories are being replayed in the modern whole-language movement. It is, in a sense, the recycling of a two-hundred-year-old idea for a new generation of educators. Goodman, a psycholinguist, trumpeted the "major shift in thinking about the reading process" represented by the holistic approach. Edelsky, Altwerger, and Flores explain their mentor's assumptions this way:

Rather than viewing reading as "getting the words," whole language educators view reading as essentially a process of creating meanings. Meaning is created through a transaction with whole, meaningful texts. . . . It is a transaction, not an extraction of the meaning from the print, in the sense that the reader-created meanings are a fusion of what the reader brings and what the text offers. . . . In a transactional model, words do not have static meanings. Rather, they have meaning potentials. (1991, 32)

As the 1980s unfolded, whole language was being adopted as the correct way to teach reading in colleges of education across the land. This wholesale endorsement by American universities meant that the lion's share of teachers entering classrooms took with them a professional commitment to whole language—and an aversion to skills, especially phonics, that come along with it.

What they didn't know was that science was, even then, finding serious flaws in many whole-language assumptions. By the next decade, even as science was challenging the approach, millions of students were falling by the wayside. Countless kids of normal to high intelligence, bereft of basic reading skills, left school ill equipped to cope in an increasingly print-based economy, where the prospects for poor readers and nonreaders were getting ever grimmer. As manufacturing jobs dried up or flowed overseas, poor readers faced few opportunities beyond menial jobs, military service, or unemployment. A lot of them are sitting in prisons.

ON THE HORNS OF A FALSE DICHOTOMY

The obstinacy of whole-language advocates, in defiance of science, is clearly fed by personal observations that reinforce their beliefs, Stanovich and Stanovich (2003) suggest. As Isabel Beck, a senior scientist at the University of Pittsburgh, observed in 1996, "People keep noticing the fact that some children or perhaps many children—in any event a subset of children—especially those who grow up in print-rich environments, don't seem to need much more than a boost in learning to read than to have their questions answered and to point things out to them in the course of dealing with books and various other authentic literacy acts" (8). In a paper presented at the Reading Hall of Fame of the International Reading Association in New Orleans that year, Beck pointed out that decoding proponents are *also* fueled by personal observation. "People keep noticing the fact that some children or perhaps many children—in any event a subset of children—don't seem to figure out the alphabetic principle, let alone some of the intricacies involved, without having the system directly and systematically presented," she said in her paper, *Discovering Reading Research* (8).

Stanovich and Stanovich lament the widespread myopia that blinds educators to the "basic fact that the two observations are not mutually exclusive— one doesn't negate the other" (35). They go on to assert that "This is the type of situation for which the scientific method was invented: a situation requiring a consensual view, triangulated across differing observations by different observers" (35).

The 1990 publication of Adams's landmark study on the role of phonics instruction in beginning reading—a study commissioned by the Department of Education under a congressional directive—added a new and persuasive voice to the din of the debate. Adams calls for banishing the pendulum and blending the best of both the phonics-based and meaning-based approaches. Written text, she argues forcefully, has both form *and* function—both "method and purpose" (1990b, 424).

"It is time," Adams says, "for us to stop bickering about which is most important. To read, children must master both, and we must help them" (1990b, 424).

Two other seminal reports written by experts in a range of fields over the next decade joined the growing chorus calling for consensus. The National Research Council's 1998 report *Preventing Reading Difficulties in Young Children* (Snow, Burns, and Griffin) and the National Reading Panel report in 2000 gave new impetus to a movement to merge meaning and skills— including, but not limited to, phonics. Many schools and publishers are responding with new programs.

But across the nation, deep divisions and suspicions remain impervious to evidence. Mention that beginning readers require "direct instruction" in decoding, and many educators react as if you were advocating something every bit as cruel and backward as rapping a child's knuckles with a ruler or sitting him in the corner sporting a dunce cap—or, as teachers were taught to do in the old days, forcing left-handed kids to write with their right hand. Suggest that little kids need phonics to learn reading and people you've known for years will bristle and give you the cold shoulder ever after. Say, "Children need systematic, explicit instruction in sound-symbol relationships," and you will be accused of squelching children's higher-order thinking skills—analysis, interpretation, independent judgment. You will, in short, be tarred as a traitor to humanism, progressivism, and probably even democracy itself.

Readers do, indeed, draw meaning from text in a sort of mental tennis game, in which the author's message bounces against the reader's prior experiences and understandings in a vigorous mental volley. Yet this idea—that the point of reading is not soaking up words from a page of print but, rather, "constructing" your own meaning from the author's words—sets up a false dichotomy, the two-horned dilemma upon which reading instruction has been skewered for centuries. Readers do interact with the author's message, imbuing the text with their singular understanding. But before the reader can do this, he must, like a World War II code breaker, decipher the jots and squiggles and lines and circles stamped upon the page.

Skills and meaning have been ripped apart in a wrong-headed belief that you can have one without the other. Just as you can't separate the mind from the brain (there is no thinking, no reasoning, no awareness, without gray matter and synaptic connections), you can't separate the letters from the words, or the words from the meaning (there is no understanding, no comprehension, no interpretation—in short, no reading—without the inked symbols pressed upon a solid surface). If you can't read the words, you can't construct any meaning. Yet the constructivists have mostly ignored word-recognition skills, as though a reader could somehow take a magical mental leap over the words straight to the meaning. Goodman, the acknowledged guru of whole language, scoffs at approaches that view "words as the key units in learning to read and write" (1986, 35).

On the other hand, some phonics advocates see reading as a mainly mechanical process, as if sounding out were an end in itself. As if a child would curl up with a pack of flash cards on a rainy Saturday afternoon. As if a worksheet were a fine substitute for a plunge into Scott O'Dell's *Island of the Blue Dolphins* or *Treasure Island* by Robert Louis Stevenson.

The truth lies between these two extremes.

Phonics as Political Football

The biggest hindrance to forward motion is the political branding of phonics. Instead of being seen simply as an approach to reading instruction, phonics has become emblematic of unprogressive teaching. Rather than being understood as a strategy for deciphering the alphabetic system—for breaking the code encrypted in print—phonics has become a watchword for backwardness in education.

The reading wars are the result of what E. D. Hirsch Jr. terms a "premature polarity" (2001, 22). Pointing out that these polarities are rife in the field of education, he defines them as "the habitual, almost automatic taking of sides on educational issues based on whether one considers oneself to be a liberal or a conservative in politics" (2001, 22). In the reading wars, he says, this polarization "has caused phonics to be viewed as an agency of right-wing suppression that deprives reading of its naturalness and impairs love of literature. 'Whole language' on the other hand, is attacked as a left-wing abandonment of adult responsibility" (2001, 22).

A Google search for the key words "phonics + 'right wing'" generates thousands of hits, giving instant credence to the fusion of these ideas in popular culture today. Anti-phonics forces have come to identify phonics with the kind of thinking that wants to censor Harry Potter books because they're about the occult. Or that forbids the teaching of contraception. Or that insists on daily recitation of the Pledge of Allegiance. Phonics proponents are tarred with the brush of archconservatism, or accused of being the henchmen of neoconservative politicians, Bible-thumping preachers, and back-to-basics zealots. In the minds of many mainstream American educators today, phonics and right-wing politics go together like shoes and socks. Researchers advocating phonics are branded as "Bushies" (even though their studies began decades before the George W. Bush administration was even a twinkle in his father's eye).

And indeed, the right wing is solidly in the phonics camp. Conservative activist Phyllis Shlafly, founder of the "pro-family" Eagle Forum, is an outspoken proponent of phonics and author of a book called *Turbo Reader*. In a 1999 column calling for schools to "scrap the failed method called whole language," Shlafly goes on to predict that they "aren't going to do that because their teachers are brainwashed into believing that phonics is a Far Right religious and political conspiracy." She adds, "How sad" (1999).

The present authors are as likely to agree with Shlafly on social and political issues as a neo-Nazi skinhead is to organize a fund-raiser for African AIDS victims. But on phonics, we have to admit that we're in sync with Shlafly, who is infamous for her ten-year battle to defeat the Equal Rights Amendment for women.

In her column titled, facetiously, "Beware of the Phonics Conspiracy," Shlafly takes issue with the left-wing insistence that phonics is part of a "vast right-wing conspiracy." She cites a 1994 college textbook for prospective teachers that raises an ominous alarm about the Far Right's "hidden agenda" of squelching independent thinking and promoting "docility and obedience

on the part of the lower classes." The textbook that makes these claims—
Reading Process and Practice: From Socio-Psycholinguistics to Whole Language, written by Goodman acolyte Constance Weaver and published by
Heinemann—devotes a humongous, twelve-square-inch paragraph to listing
"major Far Right leaders and groups." Shlafly is on the list, along with tele-
vangelists Rev. Jerry Falwell of the Moral Majority and Rev. Pat Robertson
of the Christian Coalition. The implication, though left unspoken, is that this
list "outs" these phonics conspirators. Yet in the very next paragraph, Weaver
backpedals fast and furiously: "Of course, it's important to note at the outset
that by no means all members of the religious or political Far Right share an
interest in promoting extensive and intensive phonics," she hedges. "Never-
theless, there is considerable agreement among at least some of the aforemen-
tioned leaders and political action groups they have founded to control what
will and won't be taught in schools" (1994, 296).

In the section titled "The Hidden Agenda of Extensive, Intensive Phonics," Weaver makes the claim that "it is not reading researchers or educators"
who advocate the explicit, systematic teaching of phonics. Rather, she
asserts, most phonics proponents are "laypersons" from the "political and
religious Far Right" (1994, 294–95). She next poses a rhetorical question:
"What motivates such advocacy?" and then follows up with this answer:
"Oddly enough, it may not necessarily be what proponents claim: namely,
the desire to teach all children to read. A great deal of the force behind such
advocacy seems to be a desire to promote a religious agenda and/or to maintain the economic status quo" (1994, 295).

Weaver's accusation—that a phonics-frenzied camp of rabid right-wingers
nefariously seeks to "maintain the socioeconomic status quo" and preserve
"socioeconomic stratification"—does smell strongly of conspiracy theory, as
Shlafly argues in her column. It also brings up one of the rank ironies of
the reading debate. That's because, as Shlafly observes, it's actually whole
language (which favors middle-class kids) that discriminates against disadvantaged children, thus shutting them out of the literacy society.

"The fact is," Shlafly writes,

> that nothing, nothing at all, has done more to prevent the "lower classes" from rising
> above their "socioeconomic stratification" than the failure to teach them how to
> read. Illiteracy is the systemic disease of the unemployed, the welfare class, and the
> prison population, all those pathetic thousands of Americans who, despite having
> attended public schools, are unable to "write my name" or "write the date." (1999)

Weaver bases her somewhat hysterical accusations on a few scattered
shreds of flimsy speculation. The only concrete evidence she offers to support
her sweeping charges is a 1986 pamphlet written by a guy named James A.

Chapman (who, by the way, wasn't significant enough in stature to make even Weaver's own list of important right-wingers). Chapman, an author of grammar and composition textbooks for Christian schools, teaches freshman English at Florida's 4,000-student Pensacola Christian College. In his pamphlet "Why Not Teach Intensive Phonics?" his arguments range from secular and supportable ("whenever initial emphasis is placed upon meaning instead of identifying the exact words that are on the page, a student is implicitly learning that individual words are not important") to religiously radical ("Christians . . . who are training young people to respond to Jesus' command to 'live by every word that proceedeth out of the mouth of God' [Matt. 4:4] should reject a system of reading that trains students to guess at words and to be content with approximate meanings") (Weaver 1994, 296). Yet once again, Weaver weasels. On the question of just how widespread such attitudes are, she prefaces the Chapman quote with the disclaimer, "Of course, Chapman does not necessarily represent the views of most Christians" (296).

To cite the writings of an obscure and unrepresentative Christian educator as proof of a vast religious cabal seeking to foist phonics on children for sinister motives is, we submit, not only misleading but also unethical. To the eight pages Weaver commits to railing against the "Far Right," she gives just a single page to the topic, "Research Supporting the Systematic Teaching of Phonics," essentially flicking off an entire body of evidence. Furthermore, following her fourteen-page discussion titled "Research Supporting a Whole Language Alternative," in which she describes findings from eight studies, Weaver waffles yet again. "The research described above," she cautions, "is a fairly small research base, and these studies are doubtless not without their limitations and flaws" (1994, 323).

On the whole, conservatives have been every bit as bilious in their condemnation of whole-language advocates as left-leaning educators like Weaver are in their vitriol against phonics proponents like Shlafly. Charges of subversive motives flow from the Right as well as from the Left. One archconservative Web publication, for example, accuses the whole-language camp of having a "socialist agenda." In a 1999 posting of WorldNetDaily, Samuel L. Blumenfeld proclaims that "the Left wants to use reading instruction as a tool of socialist indoctrination" (1999). Some Christian groups—adherents to the same brand of fundamentalism as Chapman's—argue that because whole language encourages readers to apply their own interpretations to written works, students of the Holy Bible might be tempted to see symbolism or nuance in the Word of God rather than literal truth.

Weaver, a professor of English at Western Michigan University, hits this idea hard in her textbook. She argues that the fetish for "getting the words 'right'" and the related obsession with "so-called literal recall" comes from the Religious Right's belief that "neither church nor parental authority nor the authority of the Scriptures is to be questioned." These authoritarian leanings lead religious fundamentalists to "promote forms of instruction that require adherence to a prescribed and thought-limiting curriculum" and to blast whole-language teachers for "promoting Godlessness" because their approach "insists that individual interpretation of texts is not only permissible but inevitable," Weaver writes (1994, 296–97).

Weaver's book, published first in 1988 and again in 1994 and 2002, has sold nearly 90,000 copies over its three editions, according to Heinemann's sales records. That a mainstream educational publisher would disseminate such brazenly political, highly prejudicial polemics, masquerading as scholarship, in a college textbook is alarming at best. Her inflammatory rhetoric and indiscriminate indictment of phonics proponents has the effect of drowning out the voices of science, research, reason, logic, scholarship, and evidence. Lost is any chance of fact-based consensus.

Hirsch, that tireless appellant for reasoned debate, laments that this kind of ideological stand-taking "not only brings investigation to an end but also tends to replace thought" (2001, 22).

Limits of Constructivism

Research tells us that reading is a synthesis of mechanics and meaning—of, as Adams insists, both form and function, both method and purpose. Mastering reading is not an either-or proposition. A child needs both word-identification skills *and* comprehension strategies to become a reader. It's like a waterproof raincoat and its fuzzy lining: To stay dry *and* warm, you need both.

Painting all learning with the broad brush of constructivism obscures critical elements of the reading process demonstrated by researchers. The mental process children use to read *words* is not the same mental process they use to glean (or "create") *meaning* from those words. Deciphering individual words in print, researchers have discovered, is altogether different from getting meaning from text. That is, the brain recognizes individual words in a way that is quite distinct from how the brain *understands* those words, connects them, and imbues them with meaning. Stanovich explains that word identification is a "modular" skill, while comprehension is more akin to the process of reasoning.

Shaywitz, after a decade of watching the brain activity of readers in action, has found that there are "at least two neural pathways for reading; one for slowly sounding out words, and another that is a speedier pathway for skilled reading" (2003, 78). In disabled readers, weaknesses in word identification—"what is essentially a lower-level language function"—blocks access to "higher-order language processes and to gaining meaning from text" (2003, 53).

There are two ways that these pathways to reading get blocked and, hence, two major groups of disabled readers, scientists suggest. "One, the classic dyslexic, is born with a glitch in his posterior reading systems," Shaywitz explains. "The second group seems to have developed into poor readers mainly, we speculate, as a result of experience. It may be the result of a combination of poor reading instruction in school and a disadvantaged language environment at home. In this group the wiring for the posterior reading system may have been laid down early on but never activated appropriately; the system is there, but it is not functioning properly" (2003, 85).

While the lower-level and higher-level processes at work in a reader's brain unquestionably work in tandem and build upon each other in a continuous give-and-take, they are distinct and therefore require different, but complementary, strategies in the classroom. Back in 1966, Harry Levin wrote an article titled "Reading Research: What, Why, and for Whom?" in *Elementary English*, laying out the simple notion that "reading may be broken into two broad sub-skills." He described them this way:

> The first is the skill of decoding the writing system to its associated language. English orthography is an impressive and complicated representation of the sounds of language. . . . In one form or another, the child must learn this code. Most importantly, teaching must be oriented to making access to the code completely automatic—to make the code transparent. The second rubric of component skills in reading concerns the use of the code—the written version of the language—for the many uses to which reading may be put. This category includes comprehension, reading for different levels of meaning, reading for pleasure, and so forth. By dividing the process of reading into these two very broad categories, I am not implying that one is more important than the other or that emphasizing one skill excludes the other. I am frankly at a loss to understand the furor that this essentially bland statement arouses. To say that reading is really comprehension is like saying that ice skating is really performing figure eights! (138–147)

Writes Virginia Berninger, "Currently, many preservice teacher training programs advocate philosophical approaches (e.g., constructivism that advises against explicit instruction) that are not consistent with what research in developmental science and educational science during the past three decades has shown is effective in teaching students with specific learning disabilities—namely, explicit instruction to bring language processes into conscious awareness" (2006).

Constructivism also fails to consider the widely varying purposes of reading and the vastly different kinds of texts. If you could, with an imaginary wide-angle lens, look in on your town's readers at any given moment, you might see a grandmother in her garden, dreamily perusing the poetry of William Stafford. A young dad puzzling over the instructions for assembling a tricycle. A single mom devouring a Harlequin romance while waiting for a bus. A medical student drinking her third cup of coffee while poring over an organic chemistry text. An elderly man squinting through his bifocals at the dosage for his new prescription medication. A bride-to-be scanning websites on tropical vacation destinations. A teenage boy, about to embark on his first date, sweating and searching for a movie review in the arts-and-entertainment section. An environmental activist scrutinizing a Forest Service study on spotted owl habitat. An executive analyzing the annual report of a rival corporation. A first-time voter scouring the voter's pamphlet for details on a series of complex ballot measures.

Your neighbors and fellow citizens are reading labels on pesticides, household chemicals, lawn fertilizers, once-a-month dog wormers, vitamin supplements, and baby formulas. They're reading menus at the corner steakhouse and the downtown sushi bar. They're studying road signs on the freeway and maps to the light-rail system. They're figuring out loan applications, job applications, bank statements, rental agreements, divorce settlements, and subpoenas.

In this rich conglomerate of reading materials, the one place where "creating" meanings makes some sense as a strategy is literature. Certainly, the evocative texts of Iris Murdoch or Ernest Hemingway invite the reader to embellish and edit, extrapolate and postulate. But there are millions upon millions of printed words in our classrooms, workplaces, and communities that need to be understood exactly as the author intended—messages without nuance whose words are meant to be read with precision and clarity. Keith Stanovich of the Ontario Institute for Studies in Education offers a simple example: "In case of fire, pull the red handle and close all doors." And this: "Send the package to Toledo, Ohio, by Federal Express" (1994, 270).

Printed messages range along a continuum from vagueness to directness, with a free-verse poem at one end and a railroad-crossing warning sign on the other. Stanovich argues that lumping all kinds of texts into one amorphous clump obscures the incredible variety of reasons people read.

A reading strategy that, at least marginally, makes sense for poems or novels can be the kiss of death for a student cramming for a biology final. Learning about, say, mitochondria or DNA requires a literal understanding of fact-based information. A student swimming in an alphabet soup of unfamiliar words and foreign concepts won't be able to latch on to "context" as a life raft. The guessing strategy that worked in second grade, when the text was a comfy storybook full of everyday words, simply can't hold the weight of technical language and complex information. Because the vocabulary of biology is unique to the field and not likely to be part of a student's general lexicon, the whole-language strategies of guessing from context or extrapolating from previous knowledge will leave the student intellectually stranded.

Stanovich concedes that the "domain of imaginative fiction" might indeed be an appropriate place for readers to create their own meanings—an approach to reading that Beers (1987) calls "an interpretive activity having little to do with the author's intentions" (374). But reading the works of novelists such as Toni Morrison or Barbara Kingsolver or, for that matter, Stephen King, represents "only a small proportion of the actual reading taking place among the general population." Says Stanovich,

> Most reading is of mundane, expository material where misreading . . . has many real negative consequences. In the natural ecology in which most reading takes place, text interpretations are highly constrained. For example, when our physicians consult a medical volume in the course of our treatment, most of us are hoping that his or her processing will not be constrained by an unrestrained constructivism whereby meanings are imposed on the information in the text. We wish the same thing when obtaining advice about legal documents, or when our auto mechanic orders a part for us. (1994, 270)

In other words, medical books, law books, and parts manuals present precise, factual information about diseases and their treatments, court cases and their resolutions, and automobile parts and their installation.

That is not to say that the doctor, lawyer, or mechanic will not bring her own expertise to bear on any decisions she makes based upon that information. And it is not to say that her individual judgment won't lead her to reach a conclusion different from that of a colleague about how the information should be used. But before she can reach a conclusion that is legitimate, ethical, and competent, she must accurately read the words on the page, *all* the words, literally and precisely. Without the core knowledge that underpins a field of study, a practitioner cannot make a valid professional judgment as to a course of action. Getting the "gist" of a complex legal case or a drug interaction study or a brake installation procedure, while failing to grasp critical details, could result in an imprisoned client, a brain-dead patient, or an injured driver. Yet whole language insists that word-level accuracy in reading is a false—even dangerous—target for young readers. It hints that no "objective reality" or body of agreed-upon factual information exists in the realm of human knowledge, only the reader's "sense" or "interpretation" of that knowledge.

Goodman maintains that words don't have meanings, they have "meaning potentials." That statement would come as a shock to Philip Babcock Gove, editor of the unabridged *Webster's Third New International Dictionary.* Amazon.com describes this leviathan of lexicography this way:

> Weighing 12.5 pounds and measuring four inches thick, its 2,662 pages define more than 450,000 words spanning "a" to "zyzzogeton," including words ("disselboom" for instance) not found in other dictionaries, plus clear definitions, comprehensive etymologies, interesting asides, literary usage quotes, and a comfortable typeface. More than 150 years of accumulated scholarship helped collect the 10,000,000 usage examples that accurately provide definitions, and $3,500,000 went into producing this impressive volume.

THE WRITER'S ART

It's worthwhile to think about literature, too, from the perspective of individual words. Educators who promote a whole-language approach are passionate about "authentic texts," especially those texts that have literary merit. American literary icon Ernest Hemingway was famous for sometimes penning only a single paragraph after an entire day holed up in a Paris bistro with his notepad. His manuscripts show countless cross-outs and inserts and words tucked sideways into the margins, a graphic record of his internal thought process. He was struggling, not just with big meanings, but with minutiae. He sweated over every word, every nuance.

Or take another genius of American fiction, Mark Twain. In an author's note to his masterpiece *The Adventures of Huckleberry Finn,* he explains the subtle but important differences in his portrayal of the many dialects his characters speak—differences that hinge on small variations in words and grammar. Twain agonized over every utterance of the runaways Huck and Jim, the fraudulent King and Duke, the feuding families of Shepherdsons and Grangerfords, and the other Mississippi River folk who people his tale. "In this book," Twain wrote in an author's note titled "Explanatory",

> a number of dialects are used, to wit: the Missouri Negro dialect; the extremest form of the backwoods Southwestern dialect; the ordinary "Pike County" dialect; and four modified varieties of this last. The shadings have not been done in a haphazard fashion, or by guesswork; but painstakingly. . . . I make this explanation for the reason that without it many readers would suppose that all these characters were trying to talk alike and not succeeding. (1884)

It's interesting to note that Goodman cites this very passage in his monograph to make the point that "people who speak differently are not deficient in any linguistic sense" and teachers should not, therefore, be hung up on "correct" forms of grammar, usage, and spelling. The irony here is that according to Goodman's notion of reading, in which the precise words don't matter, Twain wasted his time fussing with those subtleties of dialect. They would be completely lost on the reader who uses the guess-and-go approach.

Or consider England's Iris Murdoch. This novelist was legendary for refusing to let her editors touch one word of the manuscripts she hand-delivered to her publisher.

All of these brilliant writers agonized over individual words as if each were a priceless treasure. They are, no doubt, spinning furiously in their graves to hear teachers tell students that the exact words don't matter: "Just get the gist, kids." As though, even if the gist were sufficient, it could somehow be divorced from the words. Goodman himself inadvertently admits that children really long to master not just the general idea of a text, but the precise details. He blithely soothes teachers' anxieties when he warns, "Teachers must expect some setbacks and even some trauma as learners struggle with themselves to accept that getting the gist of what they are reading is more important than getting each word right" (1986, 57).

Goodman follower Edelsky and her coauthors explain that language systems "offer clues to narrow down the possibilities" of which words might fit in any given context. Based on these semantic clues, then, readers "predict words, sentence types, meanings, and so on" (1991, 12). The authors give this example: "If *she should* precedes *thr*, cues from the syntactic system help readers predict *throw* rather than *three*." Sure. But having a somewhat narrower panoply of possibilities fails, in the end, to nail the word—and, ultimately, the meaning. Using Edelsky's three-letter clue, a reader might come up with the following possibilities besides *she should throw*: *she should thrash, she should thread, she should thrust, she should thrive,* or *she should threaten.*

The modicum of predictability that narrative text offers to guide the reader dissolves quite completely in the imaginative ether of verse. It is, in fact, its very *unpredictability*—the semantic surprises, the startling images, the waywardness of wording—that gives poetry its power and allure. A reader who has been taught to depend on predictability and context will be like a hummingbird flying in a hurricane. Consider these lines from Robert Frost's "Design" (1949, 396):

> What had that flower to do with being white,
> The wayside blue and innocent heal-all?
> What brought the kindred spider to that height,
> Then steered the white moth thither in the night?
> What but design of darkness to appall?—
> If design govern in a thing so small.

Or imagine trying to use guesswork to make sense of Shakespeare's Sonnet 18, which begins, "Shall I compare thee to a summer's day?" made all the muddier by the archaic lingo of the Renaissance. Here are a few lines:

> Rough winds do shake the darling buds of May,
> And summer's lease hath all too short a date:
> Sometime too hot the eye of heaven shines,
> And often is his gold complexion dimm'd;
> And every fair from fair sometime declines,
> By chance, or nature's changing course, untrimm'd. (Booth 1977, 19)

The predictability premise becomes even shakier when it comes to free verse, where not even the promise of a rhyme provides a hint for a guess. Imagine how far the predict-and-guess strategy would get you in Kilian McDonnell's poem "The Monks of St. John's File in for Prayer" (2003). Consider these lines:

> In we shuffle, hooded amplitudes,
> scapulared brooms, a stray earring, skin-heads
> and flowing locks, blind in one eye,
> hooked-nosed, handsome as a prince
> (and knows it), a five-thumbed organist,
> an acolyte who sings in quarter tones,
> one slightly swollen keeper of the bees,
> the carpenter minus a finger here and there.

We wonder, too, how any reader, trained to guess her way through text based on "context" and the "predictability" of language, would fare with the writings of neurologist Oliver Sacks, whose best-selling books about the quirky vagaries of brain-based disorders such as Parkinson's disease and Tourette's syndrome brim with human pathos, scientific lingo, and the most unexpected events. In his collection of case studies called *An Anthropologist on Mars*, for example, Sacks writes with great warmth and wonder about a Canadian surgeon's weird and endearing tics, including an obsessive attraction to odd and resonant names, which the Touretter blurts from time to time. The surgeon's odd-name list, Sacks writes, begins with Oginga Odinga, "with its alliterations," and "contains more than 200 names." He goes on:

Of these, twenty-two are "current"—apt to be regurgitated at any moment and chewed over, repeated, and savored internally. Of the twenty-two, the name of Slavek J. Hurka—an industrial-relations professor at the University of Saskatchewan . . .—goes the furthest back; it started to echolate itself in 1974. . . . Most words last only a few months. Some of the names (Boris Blank, Floyd Flake,

:ris Gook, Lubor J. Zink) have a short, percussive quality. Others (Yelberton A.
le, Babaloo Mandel) are marked by euphonious polysyllabic alliterations. Echo-
a freezes sounds, arrests time, preserves stimuli as "foreign bodies" or echoes in
: mind, maintaining an alien existence, like implants. (1995, 88–89)

A passage as richly original, complex, and challenging as this one by a
gifted writer-scientist will surely elude comprehension for the hapless reader
who has never learned to decode. There is a jarring dissonance in a reading
theory that on one hand elevates and embraces "authentic texts," yet on the
other hand dismisses authors' well-chosen words, in all their precision and,
yes, their unpredictability.

More Holes in Whole Language

Whole language rests on two basic theoretical pillars: First, as we have discussed, that reading isn't actually about words. And second, that children
learn to read "naturally," in the same way that they learn to speak.

The widespread acceptance of the first notion—that specific words are
unimportant as long as you get the "gist" of the narrative—is hard to fathom.
Goodman is famous for telling *New York Times* reporter Edward B. Fiske in
1975 that it's no big deal if a child "reads" the word "pony" instead of the
word "horse" (27). He pooh-poohed the importance of such trivial distinctions. We submit that it matters a great deal whether Christopher Reeve's
mount was a horse or a pony on the day in 1995 when he fell and shattered
his spine, and that when Prince Charles and Camilla ride to the hounds,
they're not trotting along on Shetlands. In making these rash statements, we
defend our position by pointing out that a polo pony resembles a Clydesdale
about as much as a dachshund resembles a Great Dane.

When is "close" close enough? Is a moth a butterfly? Is a scone a biscuit?
Is a pansy a petunia? Is "Goodwin" close enough to "Goodman"? How
about "Gudmun"?

As Adams explains, words are the "raw data of text." She elaborates:

It is the words of a text that evoke the starter concepts and relationships from which
its meaning must be built. Research has shown that for skillful readers, and regardless of the difficulty of the text, the basic dynamic of reading is line by line, left to
right, word by word. It is because skillful readers are able to recognize words so
quickly that they can take in text at rates of approximately five words per second or
nearly a full typewritten page per minute. It is because their capacity for word recognition is so over-learned and effortless that it proceeds almost subattentionally, feed-
ing rather than competing with comprehension processes. Most surprising of all,
research has taught us that what enables this remarkably swift and efficient capacity
to recognize words is the skillful reader's deep and ready knowledge of their spell-

ings and spelling-speech correspondences. During that fraction of a second while the eyes are paused on any given word of the text, its spelling is registered with complete, letter-wise precision even as it is instantly and automatically mapped to the speech patterns it represents. (1998, 74)

The idea that a reader needn't actually identify the words on the page to get (or "create") the meaning of the text is absurd on its face. Despite such prima facie flaws in Goodman's theories, thousands of converts have lined up, like the crowd admiring the emperor's new clothes, to cheer his claims.

The popular appeal of the second notion is easier to understand. It does not seem implausible—especially if you happen to be an intuitive reader—that reading is as natural a human behavior as speaking. It is significant to note that Goodman and followers don't actually use the words "learning to read." Rather, their theory lumps speaking, reading, and writing together simply as "language." Learning to read is subsumed in the broad activity of "language learning." They then close their eyes and take a soaring theoretical leap. They argue that because written and oral language are one and the same, and because speaking is an innate ability—one that virtually every toddler masters with ease—reading, too, must be a "natural" act. But the logic is fallacious because the underlying premise is false. It has been repudiated by research on the process of reading.

The origins of oral language are as ancient as the long-buried bones of our stone-aged ancestors. Eminent linguists such as Noam Chomsky and Steven Pinker estimate that humans uttered their first words as much as a million years ago (Pinker, 1994). Speech was an evolutionary adaptation. Writing, on the other hand, appeared a mere 5,000 years ago. Print was a human invention. Writing is a representation of speech, encoded in symbols. English is an alphabetic language, which means we have symbols—twenty-six of them—to represent the sounds that our tongues make as we talk. One of the leading linguists of the twentieth century, Leonard Bloomfield, makes the distinction clear when he says, "Writing is not language, but merely a way of recording language by visible marks" (1933, 21).

Learning to speak and learning to write are as different as, say, taking your first wobbly steps and dancing Swan Lake. Or between thrumming chubby fingers on your highchair and playing a Mozart concerto on a piano. One comes without coaching; the other requires a teacher, a set of exercises, and years of practice to master. One is embedded in the genes; the other must be taught. One happens on a preconscious level; the other takes place in the conscious mind.

In their book *Whole Language: What's the Difference?* Edelsky, Altwerger, and Flores scold teachers who imagine that they're doing whole language when they teach "skills in context" or when they weave lots of rich literature into their reading programs. Such approaches, the authors chide, do not meet the lofty standards of whole language that their mentor Goodman set out in his 1986 monograph. That's because in its pure form, the whole-language classroom doesn't *have* a reading program. Students will learn to read incidentally as they engage in meaningful, "authentic" projects, the authors argue. Here's how whole-language proponent Constance Weaver enumerates the principles of whole language, which she calls a "transactional" model for reading instruction: "Reading is not taught per se: strategies are discussed as needed, while discussing literature, etc.; teacher and students discuss and try strategies in the context of authentic reading; emphasis on discussing and inviting; teacher and students may collaborate to make lists of strategies they use; teacher and students together are authorities; trust in the learner" (1994, 388).

Literature might be central to such a classroom, but not necessarily. A whole-language teacher might, instead, emphasize science projects and exclude literature. Edelsky suggests, for example, that a whole-language classroom might be one in which "children spend the whole year raising chickens and selling the eggs (including writing statements to persuade school board members that such a curriculum would be beneficial, reading advice about how to increase egg production, and writing advertisements to increase sales)" (42). Kids will be so engrossed in their poultry project, the theory goes, that they will be able to decipher agricultural bulletins and poultry-industry journals without having ever received any direct instruction in reading.

These whole-language purists scoff at basals or, for that matter, *any* materials designed to teach reading. They are equally disdainful of skills instruction, which they mock with such terms as "decoding tricks," "letter-naming tricks," and "fake writing." Their scorn is directed not only at instruction in phonemic awareness and phonics but also at activities seeking to build vocabulary, fluency, and comprehension. They dismiss these activities derisively as "exercises." Anything that is not "real" reading for a "genuine" purpose (such as raising chickens) is a fraud.

If we extend this belief to other human endeavors—sports, for instance—we would have to conclude that basketball players, rather than practicing their dunks and jump shots for hours in the gym, should instead play only "real" games. Or, in the area of music, that an oboe student shouldn't practice repetitive scales in her bedroom, nor a concert pianist rehearse a difficult fugue in an empty auditorium, because those activities are meaningless "exercises," not "authentic" experiences.

Boiled down to its essence, whole-language instruction rests on the theory that children "learn to read by reading." As in any other human endeavor, learning, practicing, and enjoyment do indeed flow, one from another, in a continuous feedback loop. No one denies that the more you read, the better you read. Yet whole language argues that skills have nothing to do with meaning—that, in fact, focusing on skills gets in the way of understanding. Current research tells us that just the opposite is true: The *lack* of skills is what blocks meaning for young readers.

Skills and meaning are, to use a tired cliché, two sides of the same coin. They are inseparable. They are equally critical in the reading process. When you watch the tortured efforts of a struggling reader, it becomes painfully obvious that without skills, that child will never discern (or create, or construct) any meaning at all. For the child staring in panic at a page of undecipherable hieroglyphs, there is no reading, no understanding, and no love of books. A Texas study found that huge numbers of kids who struggle with reading would rather clean their room than read a book. At least one little girl said scrubbing the mildew off the bathtub would be more fun than reading, researcher Connie Juel reported in that longitudinal study, published in 1988 (Adams 1990b).

Just as certainly, sounding out words without understanding them is an exercise in absurdity. As far as we know, no one—not even the most rabid phonics fan—has ever argued in favor of "sounds only" instruction.

If you accept the premise that reading is as natural as speaking, then it stands to reason that a student might need nothing more than "exposure" to print to unlock its message. But the study of linguistics and research into reading processes do not support the premise underlying the just-immerse-them-in-print approach. The brain processes print differently than it processes speech. As a human invention, writing is passed down not by our genes but by our caregivers and our teachers.

Think about another human invention, the sport of swimming. A baby's "natural" paddling behavior when held in a pool by his mother can be compared to his first gurgles and goo-goos when listening to a bedtime story. That is, babies and toddlers often exhibit instinctive swimlike behaviors without instruction. Yet we can't think of any parent who would "expose" her child to a lake or a swimming pool on the chance that the child will learn to swim "naturally."

The opening scene of the movie *The Shipping News*, based on the Pulitzer Prize–winning novel by Annie Proulx, in which the young Quoyle, submerged in all his clothes, flails wildly in a desperate, frantic effort to get a gulp of air after his father has tossed him into the water to "teach" him to swim, would fill any mother's heart with horror. Rather, she will enroll her child in lessons at the local park, summer after summer, while her little paddler builds skills as he progresses from the Goldfish class to the Penguins, Otters, Seals, Polar Bears, Dolphins, and Sharks. The four basic strokes—crawl, backstroke, breast stroke, and butterfly—are learned through direct instruction and, for competitive swimmers, countless hours of "exercises" to perfect technique, build stamina, and increase speed. U.S. gold medalist Michael Phelps clocked hundreds of hours exercising in his hometown pool for each of the few minutes he actually raced in Athens in 2004.

If someone spends a lot of time in a pool without instruction, he might be able to keep his head above water. But we've all seen the awkward splashing and flapping of an untutored swimmer, compared with the slicing glide of a skilled one. The "just-expose-'em-to-print" approach to reading instruction corresponds to the "sink-or-swim" approach to swimming instruction. When the whole-language argument that "kids learn to read by reading" is applied to swimming (that is, "kids learn to swim by swimming"), you inevitably see a lot of drowning. For every child who skims coolly to the end of the pool, there are three who are choking and sputtering in deep water, and a couple more who are dead on the bottom.

The academic equivalent happens in classrooms where reading is left to chance, to happenstance, to guesswork. The research evidence is clear: "Students are more likely to acquire decoding skills if the instructional program provides time and varied opportunities to acquire these skills," Chall says. "Some students will learn the principles on their own, but many will not in the absence of systematic training" (1983, 28).

Education professor Martin Kozloff of the University of North Carolina at Wilmington devotes a 2002 paper titled "Rhetoric and Revolution: Kenneth Goodman's Psycholinguistic Guessing Game" to exposing the "fallacies" underlying the whole-language philosophy. Kozloff is scathing when he concludes that "whole language rests on a fantasy—a dreamy way of thinking—in which there is no boundary between how we think about things and how things actually are. Once new teachers are seduced into this dream world, almost any bizarre and baseless statements can be taken as sage wisdom" (Kozloff 2002).

Kozloff puzzles over why Goodman and the ideas that "spawned the whole-language movement" were "so easily accepted" in the education community. Calling the phenomenon "an interesting sociological question," Kozloff asks, "What cultural circumstances disposed so many education students, administrators, college professors, boards of education, and veteran teachers to so easily and so thoroughly accept Goodman's psycholinguistic guess game as a premise for their reading curricula?" (2002).

Another researcher mystified by the onslaught of whole language on education is P. David Pearson. "Never have I witnessed anything like the rapid spread of the whole-language movement," he wrote in a 1989 article titled "Reading the Whole Language Movement" in the *Elementary School Journal*. "Pick your metaphor—an epidemic, wildfire, manna from heaven—whole language has spread so rapidly throughout North America that it is a fact of life in literacy curriculum and research" (231–41).

As Easy as Pie

Dorothy Blosser Whitehead, cofounder of the Blosser Center for Dyslexia Resources, thinks she has the answer to the mystery. When asked why the whole-language approach is so popular, the eighty-four-year-old reading disabilities expert shrugs and says, "Because it's easy."

Goodman's own writings support Whitehead's contention. In his 1986 monograph, Goodman argues again and again that the teaching and learning of reading are a piece of cake if you fling the basals and curriculum materials out the window (or "donate them to a paper drive," as he suggests) and turn kids loose with "real" reading materials. (Goodman's disdain for commercial reading-instruction materials seems a bit disingenuous, given his authorship of the Scott, Foresman program *Reading Unlimited*, popular in the 1970s.) The word "easy" is, for him, a mantra; he uses it at least thirty times in the space of eighty pages. The title of his very first chapter, in fact, is "Whole Language: The Easy Way to Language Development." Here's a sampling of statements:

- "If we want to keep language learning *easy*, we have to help learners learn from whole to part" (1986, 20, italics added).
- "Language development and learning through language will prosper when schools focus on what makes language *easy* to learn" (1986, 22, italics added).
- "Whole language teachers know, when they work with language that is whole and sensible, that all parts will be in proper perspective and learning will be *easy*" (1986, 28, italics added).

Certainly, the illusion that teaching reading is easy is seductive to some, just as the sellers of diet products are able to lure customers with eat-all-you-want-and-never-be-hungry promises of rapid, permanent, and painless weight loss. But as Adams says,

Useful knowledge of the spelling-to-speech correspondences of English does not come naturally. For all children, it requires a great deal of practice, and for many children, it is not easy. The acquisition of this knowledge depends on developing a reflective appreciation of the phonemic structure of the spoken language; on learning about letter-sound correspondences and spelling conventions . . . ; and on consolidating and extending this knowledge by using it in the course of one's own reading and writing. Each of these accomplishments depends, in turn, on certain insights and observations that for many if not most children are simply not forthcoming without special instructional guidance and support. (1998, 74)

There's another likely reason that whole language holds sway with so many educators: It seems to support the love of reading. Many teachers are themselves passionate readers, and the teaching of discrete skills can seem anathema to the joy of dipping into a really good story. In the summer of 2004, one of the present authors attended the first meeting of the Oregon Literacy Leadership State Steering Committee, which includes the governor, the state schools' superintendent, legislators, and educators from the local and state levels and from higher ed. As people went around the table, introducing themselves one by one, virtually every one said they wanted to participate because they "love to read" and want children to love reading, too.

Thousands of educators like these—deeply caring professionals who love kids and love books and want to share that passion with their students—have been misled by the whole-language movement. They have been taken in by the fraudulent and insupportable claim that reading is as natural and easy to learn as speaking. In a 2004 interview with Children of the Code published online, Lyon says,

Surprisingly, a lot of people will say, "Well, I never learned phonics; I learned by this or this, nobody ever taught me phonics and I read OK." We'll bring them into our laboratories and we'll have them read a sentence and put a word in there that they have never seen before, and guess what they use? Phonics. And they use it because a lot of our kids who can learn to read under any instructional method, no matter how cockamamie, are able to do that because they have already been taught these foundational building blocks. . . . When I was bringing my kids up, I read to them all the time. I read to them systematically, I pointed out letters, I pointed out sounds, I played *Twinkle, Twinkle Little Star*, Eeny Meeny Miny Mo, I read Dr. Seuss; they were inundated with all of this information that tears language apart. So their brains are now deploying neurons to tear things apart. . . . Once they get to kindergarten and first grade, a lot of our kids have these building blocks already. We've got a lot of five-year-olds who know all the letters of the alphabet, who know quite a few sounds, if not all of the sounds, and they're ready to go. They have the building blocks. And because they have them and they move on under any cockamamie approach, a lot of people think it's the cockamamie approach that's teaching them to read. And that's how a lot of this philosophy and belief gets situated. (2004)

In their genuine desire to instill love of literature in kids by withholding direct instruction in skills, teachers may be, unwittingly, achieving the opposite of their intention. At the very same time that whole language has flourished widely in America's classrooms, Americans' leisure-time reading has dropped off steeply—especially the reading of literature. An alarming study by the National Endowment for the Arts, published in June 2004, notes that during the entire year of 2002, fewer than half of Americans (46.7 percent) read even one piece of literature (including popular genres such as Westerns and mysteries). Not a bodice-buster romance, not a Reader's Digest condensed novel, not even one measly haiku. "At the current rate of loss," the report cautions, "literary reading as a leisure activity will virtually disappear in half a century" (p. xiii). The report, titled *Reading at Risk: A Survey of Literary Reading in America*, is worth quoting at length:

> Due to higher overall levels of education in America over the past 20 years and the correlation between literature participation and education, one might think that there would have been an increase in the popularity of literature since 1982. However, an analysis of the demographic characteristics of literary readers in 1982, 1992, and 2002 shows a widespread decline in the literary reading rates of people from a range of demographic backgrounds. In fact, literary reading rates decreased for men, women, all ethnic and racial groups, all education groups, and all age groups. . . . There were statistically significant decreases in literary reading for the following demographic groups: men and women, Hispanic Americans, white Americans, African Americans, people in all categories of educational attainment, and adults 18–24, whose literary reading rate dropped from 60 percent in 1982 to 43 percent in 2002—a drop of 17 percentage points. (2004, 22–23)

While the NEA implicates such culprits as television, videogames, and computers in the nation's literary skid, it goes on to note that a stunning percentage of the population "may not have been capable of reading and understanding most novels, short stories, poetry, and plays" (2004, 15). A 1995 report from the National Center for Education Statistics (NCES) shows that 45 percent of adults—nearly half of the population—read at "prose literacy levels" one and two. "People scoring at levels one and two," the NEA observes, "probably do not have the skills necessary to read many types of literature" (2004, 15).

Is it a coincidence that the percentage of Americans who are *unable* to read literature (45 percent) is nearly identical to the percentage of Americans who *don't* read literature (46.7 percent)? We suspect not.

Liberals in the Laboratory

In the research labs and colleges of education where the leading minds in reading instruction have been studying brain activity and instructional strategies for more than thirty years, the political labels and conspiracy theories hold no sway. As reported in Florida State University's newsletter *Research in Review* (Stephenson 2002), Joseph Torgesen took a survey of ten top reading scientists whose work supports systematic phonics instruction. Most of the university researchers leading the nation's pro-phonics movement are, in fact, politically liberal, the newsletter revealed.

Conservatives like to take credit for the new respectability phonics' has gained in certain quarters, most notably in the Bush White House and the 107th Congress, which passed the landmark (and deeply controversial) No Child Left Behind Act in 2001. In fact, however, whatever respectability phonics has won belongs not to ideology but to the rigors of sound science. Frank Stephenson, editor of *Research in Review*, writing about the pro-phonics stance of No Child Left Behind in the summer 2002 issue, reported that

> a leading Republican candidate for governor in Alabama bragged to a radio audience that the long overdue measure is a triumph of "right-thinking conservatives" now in power in Washington. He went on to imply that the central, "back to basics" message now being sent to schoolhouses coast to coast essentially is a product of conservative think-tanks, practically a page out of the Republican playbook. (Stephenson 2002)

What that fellow didn't realize, Stephenson notes, is that the credit was misplaced. "Conservatives can believe that all they like," he writes, "but the facts are otherwise. If the voices and hard work of a few long-suffering, liberal-minded, predominantly Democrat-leaning university researchers scattered across the nation had gone ignored, much of the 'phonics first' teeth in the Bush bill wouldn't exist" (Stephenson 2002).

Admittedly, there are some very strange bedfellows tucked up together in the pro-phonics camp. Liberal PhDs, medical doctors, and dyslexia advocacy groups such as the International Dyslexia Association are snuggled up with such conservative groups as the Foundation for Economic Education and Shlafly's Eagle Forum. Dorothy Blosser Whitehead, a consummate liberal, expresses great chagrin about finding herself on the same side as the Religious Right on this issue. "It's embarrassing," she says.

MOVEMENT FOR CONSENSUS

The new movement for consensus in reading instruction centers on the finding that skills and meaning are, quite simply, inseparable in the reading process. It's a call for an end to one-upmanship in reading, for a laying down of the "better-than" and "instead-of" arguments: skills are better than meaning, or we must teach meaning instead of skills. "In the reading wars . . . the majority of participants now say that they are in favor of a 'balanced' approach that includes phonics and good literature," Hirsch wrote in the March 2003 issue of *Principal Leadership* (21). For example, P. David Pearson, dean of the Graduate School of Education at UC Berkeley, lays out an elegant and reasoned review of reading research and politics in a paper published by the Center for the Improvement of Early Reading Achievement titled *Reading in the Twentieth Century*. Pearson (then at Michigan State University) called for an "ecologically balanced approach" (2001, 33). In a later paper, Pearson and his colleague Taffy E. Raphael elaborate on the concept:

> We borrow from environmental science the concept of "ecological balance," which suggests a system that works together to support each individual component—a curriculum that doesn't pit one aspect against another. In doing so, we hope to suggest that we must shift the debates about balance *away* from single-dimension discussions of what to teach and what not to teach, and *toward* the notion that achieving a balanced literacy curriculum is a logical goal of all literacy educators. (Pearson and Raphael)

Hirsch, optimistic about the reading wars, has seen signs that "the ideological and scientific strands, which had been fused in the hot disputes, began to be disentangled." He attributes "this happy result" to the decision by the National Institutes of Health—which he calls "the premier disinterested scientific institution in the nation"—that the "improvement of scientific knowledge about reading was of great national importance and deserved the attention of the best, most hard-headed science, free of ideological taint." That research, along with the review of research from the National Academy of Sciences and reports on the research addressed to teachers in the *American Educator*, the magazine of the American Federation of Teachers, has begun to "turn the tide of opinion," Hirsch observes in the March 2003 issue of *Principal Leadership* (21).

Despite Hirsch's optimism and some nascent signs of a truce, the furor that befuddled Levin forty years ago is still with us. For reading instruction to move forward in America, educators must find a place where phonics and progressivism, skills and humanism, aren't seen as mutually exclusive—where teachers can employ the findings of credible research without feeling they must throw out "child-centered" approaches.

But in the minds of many educators, "phonics" has an evil twin—"drill and practice" or "skill and drill," known euphemistically as "drill and kill." As long as educators think that teaching phonics means bludgeoning children with deadening drills, reading instruction cannot move forward. We once visited a back-to-basics charter school in Phoenix where little kids, buttoned up in crisp uniforms, sat tall as soldiers in ruler-straight rows, facing front, spewing out vowel sounds to the flip-flip-flip of flash cards. Lockstep. Mess up, little Caitlin, and you'll get scolded and shamed by a drill sergeant masquerading as a teacher.

This is the kind of classroom that most teachers in America would wish to encounter only in a nightmare, complete with cold sweats. This military-school approach—what Dewey calls "chain-gang and straitjacket procedures"—is what springs to the minds of many caring educators when they contemplate phonics instruction. There seems to be a belief hard-wired into the hearts of many educators that if phonics were to be an accepted strategy for teaching reading, schools would all revert to nonstop rote instruction, abandoning active learning, developmentally appropriate practices, and, most alarming, joy in the classroom.

"There's a myth," says researcher Virginia Berninger, "that explicit instruction is skill and drill, but that is not the case. The advocates of whole language and constructivism do not seem to understand that the key to scientifically supported explicit instruction involves far more than lectures, scripts, and drills." There are plenty of ways to develop linguistic awareness, she says, "in reflective ways that are intellectually engaging" (2006).

Phonics, whether taught explicitly or discovered intuitively, opens the door to skilled reading for children. Researchers have found that most children don't figure it out on their own. Rather, they need direct, systematic instruction. And for disadvantaged kids and children with biologically based learning disabilities, such instruction is, quite simply, essential.

A few children infer the process of identifying words without direct instruction, giving the illusion that the ways in which patterns of sound are mapped onto patterns of symbols don't need to be taught. Whole language is designed for this intuitive reader, the child gifted with insight into the logic and structure of written language.

Routman, noticing that good readers have a solid grasp of phonics, posits that "children learn phonics best after they can already read. I am convinced," she wrote in *Transitions*, "that the reason our good readers are good at phonics is that in their being able to read they can intuitively make sense of phonics" (1988, 44). Adams, with her usual cool-headed diplomacy, lays out Routman's argument with a polite verbal punch. Acknowledging that "Routman's observation that good readers, as a group, are quite facile with phonics is correct," she then explains that Routman has put the cart miles ahead of the horse. "Her conjecture that this is because they are good readers is just backwards," Adams asserts. "Again, scientific research argues incontrovertibly that becoming a good reader depends on understanding and using spellings and spelling-sound correspondences and, conversely, that poorly developed knowledge or facility with spellings and spelling-sound correspondences is the most pervasive cause of reading delay or disability" (1998, 86).

Aside from the prodigy, most children who read as effortlessly as they toddled or talk grew up with lots of interactive language experience with literate adults. Children, Goodman asserts, "begin to develop their competence with print in response to literacy events long before they go to school. At a very young age, children respond to books and to print in the environment and to adults reading to them" (1986, 21). He doesn't say "some" children, or "privileged" children, or children who live on quiet cul-de-sacs with golden retriever puppies and jungle gyms in their backyards. It seems clear, however, that he wasn't thinking about children who live in moldering tenements where the closest thing to a pet is the Chihuahua-sized rat nosing around the garbage in the back alley, and where the only reading material is the eviction notice nailed to the door across the hall.

This utopian view was expressed in romantic terms by Goodman's early twentieth-century soul mate Edmund Burke Huey. "All that is needed," Huey wrote in 1908, "is books of good old jingles and rhymes and folk stories and fairy tales, with illustrative pictures, and a mother or father or friend who cares enough for children to . . . read aloud to them. The [child's] . . . natural learning to read is only a question of time" (Huey 1968, 332).

Flesch, in his usual scathing tone, responds: "Huey's recipe for teaching reading is almost exactly what is being followed to this day in most of our schools. They *expect* the child to be taught by this miraculous method *at home* and are sorely disappointed if the parents leave them in the lurch. . . . The schools assume that the parents play an enormous part in teaching the small child to read, and they're consciously or unconsciously fiercely resentful when parents fall down on that unspoken contract. . . . And so the responsibility for Johnny's reading trouble is neatly placed on his parents' shoulders" (1981, 149–51).

In essence, whole language is geared for middle-class kids. To kids who go to bed with empty stomachs instead of with *Goodnight Moon* (and to kids whose brains fail to intuit the secrets of print), whole language gives a shrug and a "tough luck."

The most powerful statement we have encountered on the importance of direct instruction for beginning readers comes from an article in *Reading Teacher*. The words of Irene W. Gaskins, Linnea C. Ehri, Cheryl Cress, Colleen O'Hara, and Katharine Donnelly are simple and seem deceptively obvious. But they zero in on the essential reason that whole language doesn't work for countless kids. "First-graders who are at risk for failure in learning to read," the researchers wrote, "do not discover what teachers leave unsaid about the complexities of word learning" (1996–1997, 325). We think this point is so much at the nub of the reading controversy that it deserves to be restated, with emphasis added: "First-graders who are at risk for failure in learning to read *do not discover what teachers leave unsaid* about the complexities of word learning." In short, no amount of hanging around books will make readers of these children.

The year after this article appeared, one of the authors, Linnea Ehri, said this: "Many teachers and educators have adopted the dogma and anti-phonics sentiments of the whole-language movement without requiring evidence or exercising critical inquiry. This situation is not only anti-scientific but also anti-intellectual and hence unhealthy for teachers, students, and our society." She is "disheartened," she said, "that our work has not made schools more effective places for teaching students to read" (1998, 112).

Wildly popular whole-language author and trainer Regie Routman is one of the most influential of the educators to embrace "the dogma and anti-phonics sentiments" of the whole-language movement. In the pages of her blockbuster books, *Transitions* and *Invitations,* Routman presents the ideas that countless teachers have taken to heart. Her "attitude about the disruptiveness of phonics and its instruction is one that is very broadly held in the field," Adams notes (1998, 85).

Despite the uphill climb against deeply entrenched attitudes in the education community, Linnea Ehri sees reason for hope. "We have some great minds at work on this problem," she says. "Fortunately, the tide seems to be turning" (1998, 112).

Phonicators: The Few, the Proud

Calls for an end to the name-calling, which has at times reduced the reading debate to the level of a gangland rumble, are coming from as far away as New Zealand. Researcher Tom Nicholson of the School of Education at the University of Auckland, lamenting the "personal acrimony and personal insults" that so often spew forth in these discussions, rattles off a few of the less-than-complimentary terms that get attached to proponents of one view or the other: neoliberals, communists, pawns of the Christian Right, "miscueteers" (a slam against Goodman's term "miscue" for reading mistakes). Asks Nicholson in a plea for civility, "Do we need to describe phonics as 'thalidomide of the mind'? Do we need to describe experimental researchers as 'vampires'? Do we really need to snub or walk away from someone at a conference because they like phonics, or whole language?"

Probably the most persistent of the derogatory terms to emerge from the debate is one that elicits wicked snickers among the anti-phonics folks: phonicator. "The word sounds like an act that would be illegal in some states," one member of the listserv TAWL (Teachers Applying Whole Language) noted ("grinningly") in an online discussion in 1996.

Jeri Mackley is one teacher who was so labeled. She never wavered from her conviction that kids need phonics to become readers. Unswayed by the fads that came and went throughout her career, shrugging off the doubts of her colleagues, Mackley doggedly stuck to the belief that "you better know how to sound out some words or else you're going to be in real trouble."

Mackley took her job very much to heart. Each June, after regretfully saying goodbye and sending off her first- or second- or third-graders for summer vacation, she would take home the class photo of her latest group and tack it up in her spare bedroom. One photo eventually became thirty. When she retired from the Portland School District in the late 1990s, the Kodachrome faces of more than 1,000 little kids—many of them by then grown up with kids of their own—smiled out from her wall.

"I love children, and I just got very attached," she says, explaining why she devoted so much wall space to her former students. "Every year, I would get all these new little kids, and it was like they were *my* little kids. There are just so many needy kids out there, *really* needy. Toward the end of my career, it was getting worse—kids being raised by their grandparents because Mom is on drugs and Dad is in prison. I had one little boy who used to stay up at night waiting for his mother to come home. One night, she never came. She was murdered on her way home from a bar on Foster Boulevard."

On the very first day she stood at the door of her very first classroom, greeting the scrubbed and the scruffy, the scraggly-toothed and the skinned-kneed, the shy and the silly, the fair-skinned and the dark, she had no doubts about her mission. "I was really self-confident," she remembers. "I thought, 'Everybody's going to read in my classroom.' And you know what? Everybody read in my classroom. And I was always in culturally deprived areas."

When whole language swept into the district like a tsunami, Mackley stooped to subterfuge, teaching phonics on the sly. But she got caught. "Usually, when the principal would drop in, I'd switch to whole language—very tricky," she confesses. "But one day, I was really sick and they couldn't get a sub, so I had to work. I was teaching phonics when the principal walked in, and I was too sick to think fast enough to switch. So I just kept right on going with the lesson."

The principal rushed back to his office and drafted a letter of discipline. "He said I was not to teach phonics," she says. "But that wasn't all. Besides bawling me out about that, he told me I wasn't to teach the kids *anything*. I was to ask them what *they* wanted to learn. Now, first- , second- , and third-graders do not know what they should be learning. I mean, some of them wanted to swing by the lights. Were you going to let them do *that*?"

Mackley was "so shook-up" about the principal's reprimand that she complained to the teacher's union. The case eventually landed on the superintendent's desk. "The superintendent called up the principal and told him he couldn't write me up for teaching phonics," Mackley reports. "He said that if his own third-grader hadn't been taught phonics, he wouldn't be reading to that day."

Recently, phonics diehards like Mackley have turned the tables on the name-callers. They have taken to calling *themselves* phonicators with an in-your-face kind of pride. The best example is the group of outliers who took the daring step of forming a phonics special-interest group within the International Reading Association—long a fierce bastion of the whole-language approach. This move might be likened to a clutch of songbirds sharing a nest with a brood of raptors. Hirsch suggests that, in fact, the phonicator slur may well have originated in the powerful 80,000-member organization. "Within the International Reading Association," he wrote in the March 2003 issue of *Principal Leadership*, "those who favored a so-called code-first approach to reading were called 'phonicators'" (21).

As a sign that the reading wars may be at least rounding a gentle bend (if not exactly turning a sharp corner) toward acceptance of phonics, Lynn Gordon, an assistant professor in the Department of Elementary Education at California State University, Northridge, was given the nod in 2002 to officially launch the phonics group. Considering the pariah status of phonics within the IRA not that long ago, Gordon's initial gathering of only a handful of members—a dozen or so souls among the 16,000 who attended the annual convention in San Francisco that first year—has a bigger significance than its size might suggest. The phonics enthusiasts may have comprised a paltry .075 percent of the reading behemoth—a barnacle on the belly of a whale—but there they were.

The group even caught the attention of the education press. "Reading Association Recognizes 'Phonicators' Group" blazed the headline in *Education Week* on May 15, 2002. The newspaper reported that the slang term got "an icy reception" from some IRA officials, who saw it as "derogatory." Gordon, however, was quoted as saying that "many phonics proponents, including herself, refer to it fondly." The education professor not only confessed to being a no-apologies phonicator, she even liked the suggestive implications of the word. "It sounds kind of naughty," she told the reporter. In fact, Gordon has submitted the term for consideration to no less a pillar of correct usage than the *Oxford English Dictionary*, according to the premiere issue of the *Phonics Bulletin* put out by the IRA Phonics Special Interest Group (2003).

"I'm not sure who originated the term," Gordon told us, "but the first time

I heard it was at a conference lecture. John Shefelbine, a wonderful reading professor at California State University, Sacramento, used it to describe himself (or perhaps he reported that he'd been accused of being a phonicator). In any case, he got a big laugh. I do fancy this neologism and, as a hobby, have kept a small collection of usages of the term in print."

Noting that "the political climate has changed in recent years," which she attributes to the combined effect of Marilyn Adam's *Beginning to Read: Thinking and Learning about Print*, the National Reading Panel report, and the bipartisan Reading First and No Child Left Behind federal legislation, "Phonics is back in, at least officially," Gordon says. "It feels like phonics fans don't have to lurk nervously in the shadows anymore, so we're comfortable enough to poke fun at ourselves. There are many instances down through history where a previously derogatory term has come to be embraced by a culture or ethnic group and I think that is what has happened here."

The phonics group membership has, if not exactly exploded, at least multiplied a bit, now standing at 100. Says Gordon, "Many newer teachers and veteran teachers, especially those teaching in the primary grades, are experiencing phonics for the first time and are finding that phonics is not bad (as some had been taught), but good (in the right doses and when taught appropriately) and simply pedagogically commonsensical."

We asked Gordon whether she had seen an "about-face" in the International Reading Association. "Well," she says,

the IRA accepted our Phonics Special Interest Group proposal four years ago, and that was exciting and wonderful for our members. We were and are delighted to have official IRA recognition and an annual venue where we would be welcome to share our expertise in this area with other reading professionals. I don't think we can feel too terribly marginalized by IRA, therefore, but I do know there are some IRA members who criticize the organization for dragging their collective feet politically and not getting on the reading-reform bandwagon more wholeheartedly. Some gripe that IRA leaders have had a bias for many years against selecting conference proposals that have phonics in the title, and a bias against publishing articles or books that promote systematic explicit phonics instruction. Personally, I do wish that they would add the word 'phonics' to the reading-topic interest list that appears on the annual IRA card that members complete when sending in dues. I would also like to see 'phonics' as a search category on the online convention program search engine on the reading.org website.

Gordon concludes with this: "I think it would be fair to say that the culture of the International Reading Association is changing, albeit slowly. When Reid Lyon spoke, by invitation, at the annual IRA convention a couple of years ago, he was warmly introduced by IRA president Leslie Morrow, who urged the audience to listen carefully to what he would be discussing. When he was done, he actually received a standing ovation by many (but not all) members. It was an extremely gratifying moment for the phonicators in the room!"

GLOSSARY OF TERMS:
DIRECT INSTRUCTION IN READING

Beginning nearly eighty years ago, researchers and practitioners have worked to devise methods for teaching language skills to dyslexic children and adults. Among the most widely known approaches are these:

- *Corrective Reading.* An intervention program for students in fourth through twelfth grades who lag behind in their reading skills. It is highly structured and sequenced and is appropriate for use with general and special education students in small groups. Authors are Susan Hanner, Gary Johnson, and Siegfried Engelmann. Resources for further study include Corrective Reading Research (www.sraonline.com) and the Florida Center for Reading Research (www.ferr.org).
- *DIBELS (Dynamic Indicators of Basic Early Reading Skills).* A set of standardized assessments developed to measure and monitor prereading and early reading subskills, including phonological awareness, alphabetic understanding, automaticity, and fluency. Each measure has been thoroughly researched and found to be predictive of later reading proficiency. The results can also be used to provide feedback for the development of individualized reading instruction objectives. DIBELS materials are free and can be downloaded from the Internet or purchased in printed form through Sopris West. Resources for further study include the DIBELS home page http://dibels.uoregon.edu/ and Sopris West http://dibelssassessment.com/.
- *Direct Instruction/DISTAR.* Direct instruction is a general term used for teaching approaches that are both teacher directed and highly interactive. Lessons are explicit and sequenced. Skills are broken into teachable subskills that are incrementally complex. DISTAR (Direct Instruction System for Teaching and Remediation), a phonics-based reading program, was developed by Siegfried Engelmann in the 1960s, primarily to help students from low-income families who lagged behind their peers in language skills. Studies for Project Follow Through, a component of Lyndon Johnson's War on Poverty, found DISTAR to be a successful school-improvement model for increasing student achievement. Resources for further study include an article titled "What Was that

Project Follow Through?" in *Effective School Practices* 15, no. 1 (Association for Direct Instruction, 1995–1996) B; Association for Direct Instruction (www.adihome.org); and Science Research Associates (SRA; www.sraonline.com).

- *Multisensory.* Methods that approach teaching simultaneously through the visual, auditory, and kinesthetic-tactile senses. For example, reading teachers using this approach link the sound of a letter with the written symbol, so that the student gets the "feeling" of how the letter is formed by tracing or copying. First used by Samuel Orton (see "Orton-Gillingham," below) and his colleagues in the 1920s, multisensory methods are reinforced with direct, explicit, sequential teaching of the structure of written English. Resources for further study include IMSLEC (the International Multisensory Structured Language Educational Council; www.imslec.org/); Fact Sheet #69-01/00, International Dyslexia Association (www.interdys.org); J. R. Birsh, ed., *Multisensory Teaching of Basic Language Skills* (Baltimore, Md.: Paul H. Brookes Publishing Co., 1999)

- *Open Court.* A core reading program written by Marilyn Adams and published by SRA. This research-based program teaches phonemic awareness, phonics, word knowledge, comprehension, writing, and language skills through explicit, systematic instruction. Resources for further study include: Research Base for Open Court (www.sraonline.com); University of Oregon, Big Ideas in Beginning Reading, Review of Comprehensive Reading Programs (http://reading.uoregon.edu/curricula/or_rfc_review_2.php).

- *Orton-Gillingham.* Developed by neuropsychiatrist Samuel Orton and educator Anna Gillingham, beginning with Orton's studies of dyslexic kids in the early 1900s. The O-G approach is a structured, multisensory, language-based method that allows students to experience a high degree of success in every lesson. The method, designed for one-to-one tutoring, forms the foundation for many other approaches, including those described below. For more information, contact the academy by phone at (845) 373-8919, by e-mail at info@ortonacademy.org, or on the Web at www.ortonacademy.org.

- *Reading Mastery.* A direct-instruction core reading program that incorporates techniques for teaching both comprehension and decoding and integrating them into successful reading, written by Elaine Brunner and Siegfried Engelmann and published by SRA. Resources for further study include: Research Base for Reading Mastery (http://darkwing.uoregon.edu/~adiep/rdgtxt.htm); Reading Mastery References (http://darkwing.uoregon.edu/~adiep/rmref.htm); University of Oregon, Big

Ideas in Beginning Reading, Review of Comprehensive Reading Programs (http://reading.uoregon.edu/curricula/or_rfc_review_2.php); and C. Schieffer, N. E. Marchand-Martella, R. C. Martella, F. L. Simonsen, and K. M. Waldron-Soler, An analysis of the Reading Mastery program: Effective components and research review, *Journal of Direct Instruction* 2 (2002), 87–119.

- *Slingerland Multisensory Approach.* An adaptation for classroom use of the Orton-Gillingham method developed by Beth Slingerland, who went on to found the nonprofit Slingerland Institute for Literacy in Bellevue, Washington, where teachers are trained to "provide the specialized instruction needed for children with dyslexia to unlock the rich world of written and spoken language." For more information, contact the institute by phone at (425) 453-1190, by e-mail at mail@slingerland.org, or on the Web at www.slingerland.org.

- *Wilson Reading System.* An intervention program for students, grade three and above, who have been unsuccessful at learning to read with other reading programs. Developed in the late 1980s at the Massachusetts Center for Students with Language/Learning Disabilities, the program is based on the principles of the O-G method of multisensory, structured, sequential, systematic instruction. It includes direct teaching of phonemic awareness, phonics, vocabulary, fluency, and comprehension. The system has expanded to include materials and training for general classroom as well as small-group intervention instruction and now has programs for younger beginning readers as well as older students and adults. Resources for further study include www.wilsonlanguage.com and www.fcrr.org/FCRRReports/PDF/wilson.pdf.

"I DON'T KNOW WHY IT'S SO EMOTIONALLY CHARGED"

Dorothy Blosser Whitehead lives alone now, quietly, in the home where she raised her three children and where, over a cup of coffee long ago, she allowed a friend to persuade her to try her hand at tutoring. From her airy, '50s-style house with its spiral staircase and ornamental garden, Whitehead went on to pioneer a one-to-one tutoring program, a training institute, and a nonprofit resource center that have, over the years, helped rescue thousands of Oregon children from reading failure.

A crack x-ray tech before she had kids ("I could zero in on a gall bladder with a cone as small as a silver dollar," she boasts), Whitehead was looking for something less hazardous to her health when her friend coaxed her into

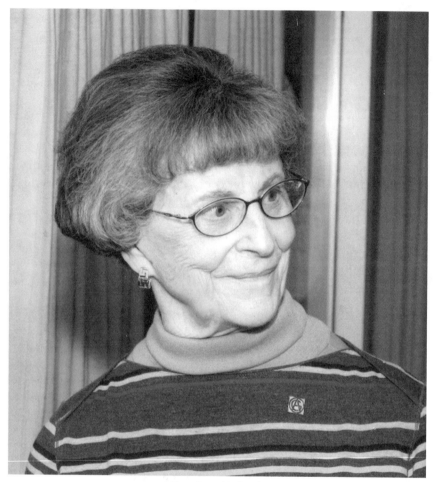

Dorothy Whitehead

taking on a struggling reader as a private pupil—a little boy named Frankie.
Only Whitehead's steely gray hair and gently aged face betray the forty-three
years that have passed since that first student sat with her, puzzling over Latin
roots and pronouncing the sounds that vowels make. That's because her mind
at eighty-three is a detailed catalog of names, faces, and conversations undi-
minished by time. She can picture it all as if it happened last week, and listening to her recount the events of the intervening decades is to be transported
along with her. Her delight over teaching Frankie to read is as effervescent
today as it was back then, when she annoyed her family by going on and on
at the dinner table, night after night, about his amazing progress.

When Whitehead went on to teach LD students in the public schools, she had the distinction of being tagged as a "phonicator." She lifts her chin with pride as she tells of being one of those phonics diehards who resisted the tectonic shift to meaning-based methods, in spite of ridicule from colleagues and flak from special-ed higher-ups. She snickers mischievously as she tells stories about her stealth tactics during the heyday of whole language, when she took to teaching phonics clandestinely, whipping out a phony whole-language lesson whenever her supervisor from the central office was spotted down the hall.

From her first teaching success with fourth-grade Frankie, Whitehead went on to train hundreds of tutors in the multisensory Orton-Gillingham method, developed by neuropsychiatrist Samuel Orton and educator Anna Gillingham early in the last century. Based on Dr. Orton's studies of dyslexic kids in the early 1900s, the method integrates the visual with the auditory and the kinesthetic. As Whitehead explains cryptically, "We teach them to read with their ears."

Whitehead founded Language Skills Therapy, Portland, Oregon; the Blosser Center for Dyslexia Resources (with Cathy Wyrick), Portland, Oregon; and Multisensory Tutor Training (with Betty Barton), a program of the Oregon Branch of the International Dyslexia Association. Her book, *Unlocking the Power of Print: A Tutor's Practicum Manual for Teaching the Dyslexic Learner*, is available at http://dyslexia.mtsu.edu/areasofinterest/psychologists/intervention/teaching.h tml).

Q: How did you become an expert in reading disability?

WHITEHEAD: It started in the late '50s, when my friend Dorothy Tyack moved to Portland. Dee was a Radcliffe graduate who'd had two years of training at the Massachusetts General Hospital Language Disorders Clinic in how to teach dyslexics. She started tutoring kids referred by a pediatrician who was practicing child psychiatry—kids who had stomach aches and didn't want to go to school. By 1959, Dee's practice had gotten too big for her to handle alone. One day, she rang my doorbell and said, "You've got to teach Frankie how to read." And I said, "I don't know how to teach reading," and she said, "Good, you'll be easier for me to train." So every week, Dee would show me how to teach a new lesson. I followed what she said, and this fourth-grade kid started to read. I couldn't believe what was happening. It was so powerful. I guess I talked about it a lot, because one night at dinner, my seven-year-old daughter said, "Mom, do we *have* to hear about Frankie tonight?"

Q: What materials were you using?

WHITEHEAD: Dee's training was all based on the Orton-Gillingham method. Our "bible" was the "big green manual" written by Samuel Orton's colleague Anna Gillingham, along with Bessie Stillwell. In those days, we had nothing but medical referrals—first from pediatricians, then from neurologists and psychologists. The phone was ringing off the wall. I said, "We have to do something about this." So we got organized, and I kept training people and we built up to twelve tutors by 1968. At first, we called ourselves "Twelve Loose Women" because nobody wanted to be in charge. The group eventually became Language Skills Therapy. We always had a tiger by the tail—never, ever feeling like we were on top of it.

Q: What is it about this type of structured approach that works so well for LD kids?

WHITEHEAD: It's multisensory. That's the key word. We don't teach them to read through their visual sense only. We also teach them through their auditory and kinesthetic senses, through hearing and writing simultaneously with seeing. That's what makes it stick. We're really teaching them to read through their ears—to hear what they're looking at. It goes right through Greek and Latin roots. Understanding of prefixes and suffixes and roots is a good way to build vocabulary.

Q: When you were working on your degree in elementary education and psychology at UC Berkeley, what were you taught about teaching reading?

WHITEHEAD: Nobody ever tried. The same thing happened when I went back to school to get my master's degree in the late 1960s. I learned about mental retardation, hard of hearing, visual impairments— wonderful stuff—but it had nothing to do with dyslexia.

Q: A lot of teachers still don't quite believe in dyslexia.

WHITEHEAD: Tell me about it. Our funniest example of this is a teacher who took our training last summer. She didn't want to come, but her special-ed director made her come. She talked all through the training and drove us nuts. At the end, she wrote on her critique, "You should not present scientific evidence as the truth." By the time I retired in 1990, whole language had come in so strong. The whole-language trainers would get up there in front of the LD teachers, all of us with master's degrees, and they would say, "Research shows . . ." and then they would spout this stuff that wasn't true. So I would go up afterwards and say, "Can you send me that research?" and they would say, "Yes." But I'd never see it. There wasn't any. It's so dishonest.

Q: Why do you think whole language has been such a phenomenon?

WHITEHEAD: It's easier. I really think the ease is a big reason. Being a classroom teacher is exhausting, and it's getting harder every year. I don't think we should ever blame teachers. They are the hardest working people in the world. But there's also this almost mystical belief in whole language.

Q: When your district adopted whole language, did it apply to special ed as well as general ed?

WHITEHEAD: Yes, whole language was mandated by the special-ed department in the district. Furthermore, they would come over to see if you were doing it. The minute they came in the building, my principal would race downstairs to protect me. I'd tell the students, "We're going to do that special lesson today." The kids always thought it was so funny. It was just all guesswork, you know.

Q: If you hit a word you can't read, just guess?

WHITEHEAD: Guess from context, guess from the pictures. My last years were very hard. They badmouthed me in the administration building. But I'm sure proud of it. It wasn't unbearable. In fact, it was kind of funny. I wasn't the only one, because there was a whole group of us who thought phonetics was important. One time, a really important educator came to the district from some big college in the Midwest. She gave a talk and called the phonics proponents "phonicators." Everybody except the phonicators fell off their chairs laughing. We just sat there, and were furious and insulted. I don't know why it's so emotionally charged. It's like religion or politics.

"I WANT THE SCIENTIFIC, I WANT THE MEASURABLE"

Judy Wright remembers trying to explain snow to a bunch of kids native to a tropical island. The closest thing in their experience was a snow cone. "To this day, I'm sure they think snow is a multicolored food," she says over a caramel latte in a crowded Northwest Portland Starbucks, talking over the whish-clank-whir of the espresso machine and the voices of *baristas* calling out coffee drinks. It was the late 1960s when Wright was a brand-new teacher in the U.S. territory of Guam, where she had to make do with out-of-date mainland textbooks full of concepts alien to her class of thirty-five third-graders. Trains were another outlandish idea to her students. For kids who had scarcely ever traveled to the far end of their tiny island, the Union Pacific was as hard to imagine as the snow-capped Cascade Mountains.

Wright, then a young wife, had to travel 6,000 miles to a speck of land in the Western Pacific to find out that she didn't know the first thing about teaching kids to read. When she followed her husband, also a teacher, to her adven-

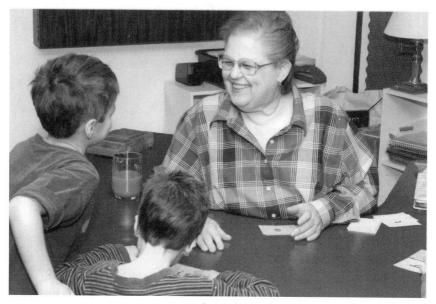

Judy Wright

turous first teaching job, the paucity of her preparation in reading instruction hadn't yet hit home. She quickly discovered that her Guamanian students, who ranged in age from seven to twelve, were mostly nonreaders. Alarmed, she felt stuck. "I realized I didn't have a clue about how to teach them to read," she recalls.

When she returned to the States, she earned a "handicapped learners" endorsement to bolster her teaching credentials, and eventually got a master's in special education. Still, she couldn't stop thinking about the hapless readers she had been unable to help on Guam. Even as her credits stacked up at Portland State University, she still wasn't learning much about how to teach reading. Then she stumbled upon a mentor. As a student teacher, she was assigned to work with the formidable Dorothy Blosser Whitehead, who was training teachers to use the multisensory Orton-Gillingham method and the reading curriculum called DISTAR, later renamed Direct Instruction. At last Wright had found what she'd been looking for ever since that first eye-opening job on Guam: the skills to get through to struggling young readers. If she hadn't met Whitehead, she says, "I'd still be searching for somebody like her."

Q: What courses on reading instruction did you take in college?
WRIGHT: I took all the required ones, but it was theory—you know, just

identifying different methods: this method does this, this method does that. There was nothing about how to actually do it.

Q: You've taught regular first-graders as well as LD kids in special-ed resource rooms. Did you use the methods you learned from Whitehead in both settings?

WRIGHT: I used DISTAR mixed with some O-G and a little bit of Recipe for Reading where you "eat" your way through the alphabet. Since I had come out of special ed, the administrators would say, "Oh, this child's having problems, put him in Judy's class." I always had a large percentage of the at-risk kids in my first-grade room. But by the end of the year, all of them could read.

Q: How did your approach fit in with the rest of the school?

WRIGHT: It didn't. It never has. The other teachers were using the basal, and I used the basal for my higher-level kids—the kids who would learn in spite of me. It doesn't make any difference what you do with those kids: They'll learn to read. But there are about 25 percent of kids who won't. You'd better really have your act together for those kids.

Q: What was the reaction of the other teachers toward your use of DIS-TAR, which has been vilified among educators for years?

WRIGHT: They'd say, "It's too structured, it's too scripted." They'd say, "I don't like teaching kids using signals." With DISTAR, the students don't respond until you give them the signal. My answer to them was, if you want to get the benefits of one-on-one instruction in a large-group setting, you have to signal their responses. Otherwise, the kids are queuing off each other. When you signal, they all respond at once and you don't get the "popcorn" effect—you know, where all sorts of responses are popping up willy-nilly and you can't tell who's getting it and who's not. In a small-group setting, you can hear if everybody is responding. DISTAR is the closest thing to one-on-one that I've ever found for a group.

Q: In your current job as the school's K–2 literacy coach, you're having all entering first-graders screened for possible placement in booster groups. What are you looking for when you screen them?

WRIGHT: The ones who have the sound-symbol correspondence pretty close are going to be OK. The ones who don't have a clue—who don't know the letter names or anything—are at risk. So we break those at-risk kids into small groups. My group is the lowest of the low—four first-graders who started the year knowing only ten or eleven letter names—no sounds, just letter names. Yesterday, right before Christmas vacation, three of the four knew all twenty-six sounds for the second day in a row. The one child who doesn't have them down yet speaks no

English—he's from Korea. He has about fourteen sounds, and I asked his teacher if I could work with him individually, just until he could get all the sounds.

Q: Why did your eyes get watery just now when you said that all those kids had mastered the letter sounds? Why is it so emotional to you?

WRIGHT: Because it's such a key to their lives. If they can't read, what can they do? Last year, one little boy named Grant had been going to the booster group, and about Thanksgiving his booster-group teacher told me, "Grant got all the sounds and all the letters!" So when I saw him, I said, 'Hey, Grant, way to go! Give me high five!' He stood up real straight and said, 'Just call me Letter Man.'"

Q: Do kids feel stigmatized by being in the booster group?

WRIGHT: I'll tell you a story about that. One day last fall, a little girl I'd never seen before showed up for the booster group. Turns out, she came on her own initiative. She "crashed" the group because she was curious about what we did. Evidently, the other students had been saying positive things about the booster group, and she didn't want to miss out.

Q: Have Oregon's state-mandated standards been a catalyst for more accountability for children's learning?

WRIGHT: Yes. One thing that came out of my special-ed training was the idea that you have to be accountable—you have to have objectives and they have to be specific and they have to be measurable. So as a special-ed teacher, I was able to say, "This child reads with 90 percent accuracy and 80 percent comprehension." I remember seeing this big book of goals for whole-language teachers, and one of the goals was, "The child will read to teacher's satisfaction." It just drove me crazy. I want the scientific, I want the measurable. Give me the facts. In general, whole-language people are not comfortable with left-brain thinking. Their idea of research is testimonials and case studies. Case studies have their place, but the problem is that you need bazillion case studies to demonstrate that a certain strategy is working in the general population rather than just in pockets. I overheard one of our district administrators saying, "Whole language is the only way to go—in your heart, you know it's right." That bothers me, because I like to know in my *head* that something's right.

Q: Whole-language proponents will argue, "Well, reading isn't about getting words."

WRIGHT: Sure, the ultimate goal of reading is comprehension. But how are you going to comprehend if you don't know what the words are? They *have* to know what the words are—the exact words, not just some guess or approximation. Close is not close enough for me. With whole language, kids are told to just skip over the word if they don't know it and say, "um" in place of the word they can't read. So the kid is reading, "Um went to the um."

Q: Did you ever hear the term "phonicator"?

WRIGHT: Yes. The district used to bring in all these speakers from New Zealand and Australia where whole language is really big. One of these presenters said, "We want to teach these children to *understand* what they're reading. We don't want them sounding out every word like the phonicators." I thought, "Oh, God, here we go again." I started calling myself The Phonicator, proudly. When I was a resource room teacher and my supervisor would come out to look at what I was doing, I made sure we did a whole-language lesson that day.

Q: One of the criticisms of direct instruction is that kids will be bored.

WRIGHT: Oh, yes, and that decodable stories like *A Pig Can Jig* are stupid because they're not literary enough. *A Pig Can Jig* is an old, old story-book, and it's based on the *-ig* word family—pig, jig, gig, big. And it *is* boring for the teacher. But the fact is that the kids are so excited to be able to read a whole page of a book. So *what* if it's a word family and all the words rhyme? They're *thrilled* with it. I think a lot of the bore-dom argument comes from an adult point of view, not from the kids' point of view.

Q: Researchers point out that kids need *both* skills and comprehension strategies.

WRIGHT: Yes, but in my district I'm very much in the minority on that—*very* much in the minority. It's an uphill battle. Mostly, it needs to change at the college and university level. It's about old dogs and new tricks. The old ideas have to die out before the new ones can take hold. But in the end, I think it gets down to an almost religious belief in one approach or another. It's very difficult to change someone's religion. A lot of the problem is that 75 percent of kids will learn to read in spite of the teacher or the method. So almost all of the teachers can feel really good about most of the kids in their room. They'll say, "You see? It works with most of the kids."

Q: What's your response to people who say that kids who don't learn to read are just unmotivated or, worse, lazy?

WRIGHT: That just sends my blood pressure up. I've never, ever met a lazy elementary school kid. If they can't read, something's getting in their way.

3

Collateral Damage: How Failed Reading Policies Hurt Kids

Children humiliated by their inability to overcome their learning problems
also tend to develop behavioral and emotional disorders. Kids with learning
problems are twice as likely to drop out of school; a disturbingly high number end up with criminal records.

—Pat Wingert and Barbara Kantrowitz
Newsweek (October 27, 1997)

Dyslexia inflicts pain. It represents a major assault on self-esteem.

—Sally Shaywitz
Overcoming Dyslexia, 2003

This chapter tells the stories of seven people with reading disabilities, all left
behind in the classroom, all scarred by the jeers and snubs of peers and by
the searing sense of shame that struggling young readers so often suffer.

But that's where their stories split apart. Of the seven LD people featured
in these pages, the four who grew up in families of means are coping pretty
well. Debra Brooks, the forty-eight-year-old daughter of a prominent rabbi,
lives with her husband and children in a lovely home in Portland's West Hills,
where she has set up a private consulting business. Edie Wyrick, the twenty-
year-old child of journalists, is majoring in philosophy and dance at the University of Oregon. Chase Spittal is an energetic eight-year-old with a private
tutor and a suburban mom who's a bulldog for his educational rights. Chuck
Arthur is running a chain of charter schools he founded to help children

become skilled readers. A first-grade teacher at Arthur Academy, Alison Post, chimes in with support for her boss's approach.

But the three from harder realities are, to borrow the lingo of an ex-con we once met, "bumpin' the bottom." Two are doing time at the Eastern Oregon Correctional Institution. The third, recently released from probation, is cleaning office buildings and trying to stay out of trouble.

The EOCI inmates, William and Dale, are both from downtrodden homes where books were even scarcer than bucks. While little Chase Spittal, with the help of his tutor, will be able to read Harry Potter by the time he's eleven or twelve, Dale was nearing forty before he learned to read well enough to tackle the J. K. Rowling series. William, too, was a nonreader until he finally cracked the alphabetic code in the medium-security prison where he and Dale are enrolled in a program for disabled learners.

The guy we're calling "Tony" was twenty-two when he learned to read at a Portland literacy program for parolees and probationers. Tony grew up with the advantage of a smart and devoted mother who did everything she could to help him learn, including hiring a tutor. But she was raising three other kids on her own in a neighborhood where the schools had a poor track record of serving their largely disadvantaged and minority students. Like Dale and William, Tony left school early, unable to unlock the meaning encoded in print.

Effective help for reading disabilities hardly ever crosses the socioeconomic divide. It's tough enough for *any* child, rich or poor, to get timely diagnosis and effective services for reading problems. But for the ones who live in trailer courts or Section 8 housing, the ones who were born to the barrios and the ghettos of America's cities or in the nation's declining blue-collar towns and its forgotten farm communities—for kids named Keisha and Maria, DeShaun and Miguel, Rusty and RaeLyn—early, targeted, effective intervention in reading is even more scarce.

"It is the concentration of poor readers in certain ethnic groups and in poor, urban neighborhoods and rural towns that is most worrisome," said the Committee on the Prevention of Reading Difficulties in Young Children in 1998 (Snow, Burns, and Griffin 1998, 98).

POISONOUS RUMORS

Biologically based reading disability cuts an indiscriminate swath across family circumstances, yet there's an illusion that dyslexia afflicts affluent kids at a higher rate than it afflicts disadvantaged kids. Very simply, that's because children who are better off more often come to the attention of schools. It's the squeaky-wheel phenomenon, common in a public education system that is increasingly strapped for staff and cash. You can't serve everyone, so you serve the kids with the most persistent parents. These affluent moms and dads, demanding services for Tucker or Taylor, Sophie or Lily, have been accused of either failing to accept their child's shortcomings gracefully or of greedily grabbing special services in an effort to give their child an unfair advantage.

This gets Sally Shaywitz's dander up. Here's what she says in *Overcoming Dyslexia*:

> The belief that somehow many parents, particularly middle-class parents living in the suburbs, are seeking a diagnosis of a learning disability to gain some imagined advantage for their child is an insidious, unfounded, and malicious rumor. These rumors poison the atmosphere and create a backlash that is harmful to children who are struggling to learn and to their parents who are struggling to understand and help them. Recently, a blue-ribbon panel concluded that rather than over-identification of suburban students as dyslexic, the problem was the relative under-identification of disadvantaged children. (2003, 338)

When it comes to reading, poor children face a host of hurdles. First, they are likely to start school with fewer literacy experiences than middle-class kids. Second, when reading troubles crop up, low-income kids are less likely than their wealthier peers to get help. The reasons are several. Their school, whether it's a crumbling brick edifice in the core of the city or a collection of mangy modules on the urban fringe, may well be short of resources and top-notch teachers. Then, too, their parents are probably unaware of the laws that mandate intervention for learning disabilities and therefore fail to make the demands that grease the wheels of special ed. Low-income parents, who are often unskilled readers themselves because of untreated dyslexia or inadequate instruction, may simply accept their child's reading problems with a sort of "chip-off-the-old-block" resignation, a fatalistic belief that the problem is a genetic inevitability. Besides, as the stories in this chapter affirm, well-heeled parents can afford to hire private tutors.

But there's another factor, an insidious attitude that festers throughout the educational system: low expectations for students from lowly circumstances. At the 2005 annual conference of the Oregon Branch of the International Dyslexia Association (ORBIDA), one educator in attendance gave voice to this attitude during a question-and-answer session. Her tone was at once challenging and defensive as she asked the presenter, "What I want to know is how can schools be expected to teach kids who come from disorganized homes where parents don't have time for their children, or where bedtime stories don't exist, or where Xboxes have replaced books?" The conference room was silent. A few people exchanged uncomfortable glances. The woman's attitude in no way reflected the collective viewpoint of ORBIDA members, mostly longtime special educators and tutors who know that such beliefs are not only misguided but also toxic to children and injurious to democratic values. The presenter took a breath and looked at the questioner. "The research tells us that we can teach any child to read," she answered. "Any child at all."

New Zealand researcher Tom Nicholson of the School of Education at University of Auckland frets about the tendency of educators to abrogate their duty to teach underprivileged kids to read. "My worry is that we will portray this problem as a social-class problem," he writes in an online paper titled *Whole Language Goes Up, Reading Standards Go Down: Fact or Fiction?* "There is certainly a 'cultural capital' difference between middle-class and low-income children. Cultural capital is part of the plot, but it is not the culprit. It would be a shame to divert attention to political issues, such as social class, when there are more proximal factors, such as ways of teaching reading, that we could look at." Nicholson takes umbrage with what he calls the "pessimistic point of view" expressed by W. Elley in the August 6, 1997, issue of the *New Zealand Education Review*: "Children who are hungry or unhappy will always be hard to bring up to average" (10). Although Nicholson's language is modulated and polite, you can almost hear him bristling at his keyboard as he pounds out this most egalitarian of statements: "Reading is not just for the rich. It is for everyone." He goes on to cite a quip by Australian Prime Minister John Howard from the September 24, 1997, issue of the *Australian*. "Reading is the main course of education," the prime minister reportedly said. "It is not the after-dinner mint." (Nicholson 1997, 4)

READING AS BIRTHRIGHT

When kids of meager means are let down by the schools they attend, the American Dream is, for them, a humbug, whatever version the dream might come in. One popular version is the three-bedroom ranch-style in the 'burbs, a Ford F150—fully loaded, with fog lights and mud flaps—and a family vacation at Six Flags (or, in its more upscale iteration, the McMansion in a gated subdivision, a Range Rover—equipped with dual-control heated seats and GPS tracking—and a vacation in Mazatlan). Or maybe the dream is a country cottage overgrown with wisteria and foxglove, a calico cat batting at bumblebees in the garden and a brown-eyed mongrel snoring on the porch. Or it might be an urban loft overlooking a trendy retail scene featuring an Internet café, a spa and health club, an organic food market, and an intimate bar where cocktails are served to the beat of techno music played by a live DJ.

Even what President George H. W. Bush mockingly called the "vision thing"—being able to conjure up an idea, to imagine what's possible—is cramped for the child who has never gotten lost in such classics of childhood as *Heidi, Treasure Island, The Adventures of Tom Sawyer,* and *The Secret Garden*, or those irresistible potboilers, the Nancy Drew and Hardy Boys mysteries. Children who've never pored over magazines like *National Geographic* or *Smithsonian* or *TIME for Kids* may never be able to picture a life beyond the Projects. The inner-city kid who can't read is unlikely to dream of living in a hand-hewn cabin nestled in an alpine meadow abloom with lupine and Indian paintbrush. Or a weather-beaten bungalow on the seashore. Or a three-story Victorian trimmed in gingerbread and shaded by an ancient elm. Or a houseboat lapped by the flow of a mile-wide river.

The variants of the dream are as diverse as the personalities and imaginations of the Americans who envision them. But for the nonreader, any rendition lies in someone else's future. At best, a nonreader will be mired in a menial job, maybe moonlighting at 7-Eleven to cover the electric bill, living in a beat-up apartment, and shopping at Wal-Mart. A night on the town is a burger at Jack in the Box and a plop on the sofa with a video from Blockbuster. At worst, that nonreader will wind up like William and Dale with rent-free lodging at a penal institution.

Skilled reading in America is in danger of becoming a birthright of the privileged, rather than an opportunity given to every American child. Most of the kids who "fall between the cracks" in the school system can be found at the bottom of the fissure between the right side and the wrong side of the tracks. "At a time when literacy is recognized as the key factor in the attack on poverty," Harvard's Chall wrote in 1967, "how to give children the right start is more than an academic question" (2).

Three decades later, Chall authored another book (this one written with Vicki A. Jacobs and Luke E. Baldwin) titled *The Reading Crisis: Why Poor Children Fall Behind* (1990), in which she describes a blockbuster report that hit the newsstands in 1966. The findings of the Coleman Report, a massive survey of 60,000 children and 4,000 schools, had "perhaps the greatest impact on educating low-income children" during the decade, Chall says. James Coleman, a sociologist at Johns Hopkins University, found that the main determinant of children's verbal achievement was family background. Largely ignored, however, was the additional finding that schools can do a great deal to mitigate the ill effects of an inadequate home. "Although several of the specific findings pointed to the powerful impact of schools and teachers on the academic development of the lower achievers and minority children,"

Chall points out, "educators and policymakers generally interpreted the findings to mean that the student's home background, rather than the school, was the primary influence on school achievement" (Chall, Jacobs, and Baldwin 1990, 2).

The Committee on the Prevention of Reading Difficulties in Young Children concurs with Chall's interpretation. Citing the congressionally mandated Prospects study of the late 1990s, which found that the gap in reading scores between middle-class and low-SES schools widened significantly between first and third grades, the committee reports, "Children living in high-poverty areas tended to fall further behind, *regardless of their initial reading level*" (Snow, Burns, and Griffin 1998, 98, italics added). Echoing Chall, the committee notes that although the Prospects findings replicated the Coleman findings in certain respects, the researchers discovered through deeper analyses of the data that "such differences *were not inevitable* (italics added)" (Snow, Burns, and Griffin 1998, 98).

The Coleman Report, despite these caveats, has become a handy rationale for schools seeking to explain low reading scores among disadvantaged groups. One member of the National Reading Panel captures that attitude in her "Minority View" statement in the panel's report (2000). As the lone dissenter among the fourteen panel members, Joanne Yatvin, an administrator in the Oregon Trail School District of Sandy, Oregon, criticized the majority, which she felt presented a narrow and biased review of existing research on reading ("irrelevant" was one of the adjectives she used to describe the report). Complaining that the findings would be of value mainly to "experimental researchers" rather than front-line educators, Yatvin pointed to what she saw as their major failing: "They do not touch on early learning and home support for literacy, matters which many experts believe are *the critical determinants of school success or failure*" (National Reading Panel 2000, 2, italics added).

In a letter to the panel accompanying her dissent, Yatvin said she had resolved to submit her minority opinion after talking with teachers at an Oregon Reading Association conference who hoped that the panel's report would decrease pressure from legislators and school boards to adopt certain kinds of curriculum materials, thereby taking away teachers' "authority to decide what's best for their students" (National Reading Panel, 2000). The letter reiterated her biggest sticking point, that "the effects of home culture on children's literacy development . . . is the [area] I believe is most critical to children's school learning, and the one I could not persuade the panel to investigate."

Most Americans are sickened by the feudal caste systems in other counties that zip each baby into a social straitjacket on the day he lets out his first yowl on earth. But when schools fail to teach kids to read accurately, fluently, and with comprehension, they are effectively cementing them into the lower social strata for life. Joanne Yatvin's point that the home is the biggest influence on kids' reading is supported by research. But we know that the *next* biggest influence is schools. We also know, based on research, that disadvantaged kids and dyslexic kids can become readers right along with their more affluent, nondisabled peers—with the right kind of instruction.

Adams says this:

> Across the literature I reviewed, children's first-grade reading achievement depends most of all on how much they know about reading before they get to school. In a way, this conclusion seems disheartening; it seems to beg the American Dream. In another way, however, this conclusion is heartening. Differences in reading potential are shown not to be strongly related to poverty, handedness, dialect, gender, IQ, mental age, or any other difficult-to-alter circumstances. They are due instead to learning and experience—and specifically to learning and experience with print and print concepts. *They are due to differences that we can teach away*—provided, of course, that we have the knowledge, sensitivity, and support to do so. (1990a, 4, italics added)

It was this challenge—how to "teach away" kids' deficits in literacy experience—that the National Reading Panel concerned itself with. The question was, How can schools raise *all* boats—the leaky dinghies and the rubber rafts, right along with the cabin cruisers and the luxury yachts?

The American ideal of sky's-the-limit opportunity is nothing but a cruel illusion when the public schools pass kids on, year after year, without giving them the one non-negotiable essential for success in the twenty-first century: the ability to read.

HIGHER EDUCATION'S "DIRTY LITTLE SECRET"

College—the gateway to good pay, prestige, and participation in the promise of America—is, for poor readers, another mirage. It's not their lack of money that keeps most low-income students out of higher education, scholars have found. It's their lack of academic qualifications. Several experts discussing scholarships for poor students on National Public Radio's "Talk of the Nation" on April 15, 2004, agreed that the most immediate need for disadvantaged students is not more financial aid but better K–12 schooling, especially reading instruction.

About two-thirds of students from the top economic quartile go on to a four-year college, said NPR guest Richard Kahlenberg, a senior fellow at the

Century Foundation in Washington, D.C., and editor of *America's Untapped Resource: Low-Income Students and Higher Education*, published by the Century Foundation Press in 2003. In contrast, only about one-fifth of students in the bottom economic quartile go to four-year colleges. "The dirty little secret of higher education," Kahlenberg said, "has been that we haven't addressed economic diversity."

Middle-class kids have a leg up when it comes time to pack their gear and head to college. "Their parents' financial and social capital has given them a crucial advantage," Walter Benn Michaels, head of the English department at the University of Illinois, Chicago, told the radio audience. "As it stands now, we really have an . . . educational system which takes kids and acknowledges whatever their class position is when they enter kindergarten, and then reproduces that class position for them at the end of the . . . years they spend going to school. So you don't really want an educational system which is nothing but a tracking device for inequality in American society."

Greg Forster, senior research associate at the Manhattan Institute, concurred with his fellow NPR guests. "There is not a large population of students who are academically able to go to college who don't go for financial reasons," he told the radio audience. Forster examined data collected by the U.S. Department of Education to find out how many students have "even the minimum qualifications" to apply to college. Besides a high school diploma and certain courses on your high school transcript, he said, "you have to be literate. You have to have basic reading skills."

What Forster and his colleagues found was that of some 4 million eighteen-year-olds in 2000, about 1.3 million had the academic qualifications necessary to apply to four-year colleges. The number of students who actually started college that year was an almost identical number—1.34 million. The researchers then broke the data down by race, and found the same results for all of the racial groups—whites, blacks, Hispanics, Asians, and American Indians.

"In each case," Forster said, "the number of kids who were college-ready academically was almost the same as the number of people who started college that year." He and his colleagues had to conclude that "the main problem is that kids are not academically ready" and that "the K–12 education system is not producing a sufficient number of students who are qualified academically to even get in the door and be considered to go to college."

When Forster paused, program moderator Neal Conan joked, "Walter Benn Michaels, I heard you nodding in agreement there." Michaels said, "Yeah. Absolutely. I think that what has just been said is absolutely right and it makes the point [that] . . . the problem is not all those kids out there who, if they could just put together the money, would go to [college]. The problem is all those kids out there who are never remotely close to being in a position to apply."

Michaels concluded that "the solution has to start much, much earlier [than college scholarships]."

An analysis of national long-term-trend reading assessments reveals that only half of the nation's white seventeen-year-olds can read well enough to understand the kind of complex information that is critical to success in college and, increasingly, in the workplace, say Kati Haycock and Sandra Huang in a report for The Education Trust (2001). The numbers are even bleaker for minority seventeen-year-olds: Less than a quarter of Latinos and less than one-fifth of African Americans can read at this level. Haycock goes on to say that by age seventeen—the very age when the buzz among your buddies should be all about college applications—only about one in seventeen youths can read and glean information from specialized text, such as the science section in the local daily. Broken down, those proportions look like this: one in 12 white seventeen-year-olds, one in 50 Latino seventeen-year-olds, and one in 100 African American seventeen-year-olds.

These statistics point to a problem not limited to the disadvantaged or the disabled. A look at the numbers reveals a nationwide deficit in reading ability. A 1992 survey by the U.S. Department of Education's National Center for Education Statistics—the National Adult Literacy Survey, which measured literacy along the dimensions of prose literacy and document literacy, as well as quantitative literacy—estimated that about one-fifth of the adult population had only rudimentary reading and writing skills. That adds up to more than 40 million Americans over the age of sixteen. A subgroup in that category—roughly 4 percent of the total adult population, or about 8 million people—was unable to perform even the simplest literacy task.

To better illuminate the nation's reading-skills picture, the National Assessment of Adult Literacy breaks down reading tasks into prose reading and document reading. Here's how the survey defines prose:

> Prose refers to any written text such as editorials, news stories, poems, and fiction, and can be broken down into two types: expository and narrative prose. Expository prose consists of printed information in the form of connected sentences and longer passages that define, describe, or inform, such as newspaper stories or written instructions. Narrative prose tells a story, but is less frequently used by adults in everyday life than by school children. Literacy with prose implies that people can locate information, integrate information from various parts of a passage of text, and write new information related to the text. Prose literacy tasks vary in the difficulty of the demands they place on readers. (National Center for Education Statistics, 2003c)

According to the 1992 National Adult Literacy Survey, the prose literacy levels of respondents fell out as follows: 21 percent at prose literacy level 1;

27 percent at prose level 2; 32 percent at prose level 3; 17 percent at prose level 4; and 3 percent at prose level 5 (Kirsch, Jungeblut, and Jenkins, 17). Thus, 40 million of the 191 million adults in the country performed in the lowest level of prose literacy. Another 52 million people performed in the second-lowest level of prose literacy. Those two figures taken together, then, account for almost half (48 percent) of American adults: 92 million people fall into the two lowest levels of prose reading literacy. Middle-level readers comprised 61 million people. About 33 million people performed at the second highest level, which means that they can "integrate or synthesize multiple pieces of information, or generate new information by combining the information provided with common knowledge, when the passages are lengthy or complex or when complex inferences are needed." Only 6 million adult Americans performed at the highest level in prose literacy.

Haigler and colleagues of the National Center for Education Statistics note further that reading prose is not the only—or even the most important— literacy skill people need to navigate the modern world with success. "One important aspect of being literate in our society is possessing the knowledge and skills to process information found in documents," they write. "Reading and using documents are not only important in our personal lives, but are also a necessary part of managing a household and performing on the job. Research has shown that adults spend more time reading documents than any other type of material" (Haigler, Harlow, O'Connor, and Campbell 1994). The National Assessment of Adult Literacy goes on to define documents this way:

> Documents are short forms or graphically displayed information found in everyday life, including job applications, payroll forms, transportation schedules, maps, tables, graphs . . . , tables of contents, and indexes. Literacy with documents means that people can locate information, repeat the search as many times as needed to find all the information, integrate information from various parts of a document, and write new information as requested in appropriate places in a document. Document literacy tasks included locating a particular intersection on a street map, using a schedule to choose the appropriate bus, or entering information on an application form. (National Center for Education Statistics, 2003c)

Disturbing deficits in Americans' document literacy turned up in the 1992 survey, essentially mirroring those in prose. Just under one-fourth (23 percent) of adults surveyed were at level 1, and just over one-fourth (28 percent) of them were at level 2. In document literacy, as in prose literacy, half of Americans (51 percent) fell into the lowest two levels. About a third (31 percent) came in at level 3. The second-highest level comprised 15 percent of adults, while only 3 percent scored at the top (National Center for Education Statistics, 2003c).

Snow's committee writes:

> The educational careers of 25 to 40 percent of American children are imperiled because they do not read well enough, quickly enough, or easily enough to ensure comprehension in their content courses in middle and secondary school. Although some men and women with reading disability can and do attain significant levels of academic and occupational achievement, more typically poor readers, unless strategic interventions in reading are afforded them, fare poorly on the educational and, subsequently, the occupational ladder. Although difficult to translate into actual dollar amounts, the costs to society are probably quite high in terms of lower productivity, underemployment, mental health services, and other measures. (Snow, Burns, and Griffin 1998, 98)

When the solutions to reading disabilities don't happen early, the consequences can be much more dire than missing out on college. William and Dale are two of the extreme casualties of a system that routinely fails poor children. When they dropped out of their Oregon high schools in the 1980s, both were illiterate. While cooling their heels in the Eastern Oregon Correctional Institution a couple of decades later, both men were identified with untreated learning disabilities. The fact that these two casualties of K–12 schooling had to have the word "inmate" stamped across their blue denim shirts to finally learn to read is a twisted irony. It broke our hearts when Dale told us, "I can't thank this place enough. As far as I'm concerned, I'm happy I came here."

The report of the 1992 National Adult Literacy Survey provides an in-depth look at the reading skills of prisoners incarcerated in state and federal prisons. The project, funded by the National Center for Education Statistics within the U.S. Department of Education and administered by the Educational Testing Service, looked at nearly 1,150 inmates, randomly selected in eighty federal and state prisons. It found that 70 percent of prisoners perform in levels 1 and 2 on the prose and document scales.

Plus, "significantly more inmates than householders reported having a learning disability," wrote researchers Karl O. Haigler, Caroline Harlow, Patricia O'Connor, and Anne Campbell in the executive summary of the report, *Literacy behind Prison Walls.* "The proficiencies of inmates with a learning disability are significantly lower than those of inmates reporting most other disabilities and are also lower than those of householders reporting a learning disability" (1994).

Noting that the inmates "scored at the very low end" of the literacy scales and that "their demonstrated proficiencies indicate that they are able to perform only the most basic literacy tasks," the authors concluded, "The fact that learning disabled people are disproportionately represented in the prison population underscores the need for accommodating learning disabilities and developing methods tailored for the learning disabled in prison learning situations" (Haigler, Harlow, O'Connor, and Campbell 1994).

Better yet, those methods and accommodations should be there in elementary school.

The profiles of individuals with dyslexia featured in this chapter are presented along with the stories of some of their advocates—mothers and literacy instructors who work with offenders. Without the commitment of parents and the compassion of professionals who work with at-risk populations, the toll from reading failure would be much higher than it is.

"CHASE WAS TAUGHT TO GUESS"

After hiding out in his room for awhile, his curiosity about the photographer's digital camera at last lured eight-year-old Chase Spittal into the living room. The little boy's initial shyness about the strangers who had come to interview him and his mother was forgotten as he examined the super high-tech camera with its fancy flash attachment, all the while asking a bazillion rapid-fire questions.

By the time we were ready to get some shots, Chase was totally into a photo-op mode, posing casually in the big recliner, and eventually standing on his head for variety. When it came to getting photos of him reading with his mom, he was determined to put the best face on his reading skills. Rejecting the slender Magic Tree House book his mom picked up as a prop, he jumped up and said, "Where's that big *thick* one?" Zooming ahead at warp speed, which is his usual velocity, he ran off to find *Harry Potter and the Prisoner of Azkaban*, which he then opened randomly and pretended to read, a look of studious intensity on his face, as the camera flashed. He *pretended* because, much to Chase's chagrin, reading has eluded him even as he begins the third grade.

Kathi Spittal was becoming increasingly alarmed as her bright little boy struggled vainly to decipher print. It just didn't make sense to her that this creative, smart, energetic kid was falling farther and farther behind his classmates. Why, when he can build a Lego Spybot all by himself, does Chase get all tangled up in written words? This is a kid who will spin you a story out of thin air—complete with punchy chapter headings—about a big battle involving a 24-calibre bazooka, a giant catapult, an evil skateboarder, a sleepy scientist, and a global pursuit that ranges from Antarctica to India to

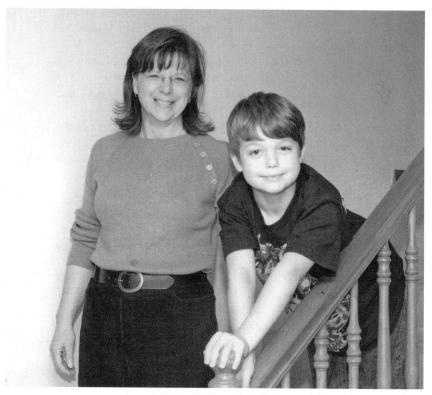

Kathi and Chase Spittal

Tokyo, Japan. Yet he can't get through a printed sentence without stumbling. "I don't read good out loud," he says, dejectedly. "I have a hard time pronouncing the words, and people say that I get them wrong."

Spittal has spent many an hour online, digging into the research on learning disabilities in an effort to obtain for Chase the help he needs. Like thousands of parents with LD kids, Spittal has found herself engaged in an increasingly nasty battle with the school district as she fights for her child's rights under the Individuals with Disabilities Education Act (IDEA).

Q: Did you have any problems learning to read as a child?
SPITTAL: No. School was easy, and reading was easy. I started checking out Big Books in the second grade. I remember vividly the day the book-mobile came to our school, and that was really exciting. I wanted to check out *The Black Stallion,* but they weren't going to let me at first. They didn't believe that a second-grader could read it and understand it.

So I started reading it out loud. They saw that I could read the text without any trouble.

Q: What was Chase like when he was a real little guy?

SPITTAL: He was brilliant from the moment he was born. [She smiles.] He's always been very, very good at picking up new words. He has a huge vocabulary, and he knows what all the words mean. Whenever I run across a new word, I'll bring it up with him and we talk about the word, he pronounces it, and if he has questions, he asks. He's really artistic and he's very spatially oriented. He's a good chess player; he beats me. I was an older mom—I had him when I was thirty-seven—and I realized when I was about six or seven months pregnant that I didn't know anything about raising a kid. So I went to the library and I took home a whole stack of books, probably two feet tall, and started reading and reading and reading. I discovered a lot of things that are so developmentally important to kids from birth to age three—you have to read to them and sing to them and talk to them all the time. I took all of that to heart, and I started doing all of those things with him when he was very young. Ever since he was really little I loved to sing the alphabet song to him. And we read all the time.

Q: When did you begin to see a problem with Chase?

SPITTAL: I started noticing that he was having trouble right away in kindergarten. He reversed letters, and he lagged behind the class in reading words. In first grade, he was in the lowest reading group and they put him in a Title I program where they read books like *The Drab Frog*.

Q: Decodable books? Books with controlled vocabulary?

SPITTAL: Yes, they're phonetic. But the students weren't taught how to sound out the words. Chase would bring these books home for me to read with him, and he would be very, very frustrated. We would figure out one word, but when he would run across the word later on in the book he couldn't remember what it was. At every parent-teacher conference when Chase was in first grade, I brought up my concerns about his reading level, about his possibly having dyslexia.

Q: What was the response?

SPITTAL: The standard answer was: "Kids develop at their own pace. It's a learning lag—he'll catch up." Only he never caught up.

Q: How did the school intervene?

SPITTAL: At my very first parent-teacher conference with Chase's second-grade teacher, she told me that she was concerned about his reading. At that point I didn't know anything about IDEA or "free-and-appropriate education" laws or IEPs. That conference really motivated me to begin looking into what was going on, what we could do.

Q: Did the school set up an evaluation for Chase?

SPITTAL: Well, they did their test for Title I, but it was just reading individual words, identifying letters and sounds, and that was it. At a meeting of Chase's student-assistance team, the resource-room teacher said, "He has a huge vocabulary. He knew most of these words. He knows all the sounds, he knows the letters; we're recommending no further action."

Q: How did you respond?

SPITTAL: Well, in the meantime, I had started doing all this research on the Web. So I said, "No, I want Chase evaluated for an IEP." It was the weirdest thing. Everything just stopped. Nobody said a word. It got real quiet. The resource-room teacher got up and left the room and came back with the permission form to evaluate him for the IEP.

Q: So essentially, you had said the magic words.

SPITTAL: Yeah. I hadn't known what words to say before I did my Web research. I had no guidance.

Q: And the school agreed to do a comprehensive evaluation by the school psychologist?

SPITTAL: Yes, but Chase lost a year.

Q: How did the evaluation come out?

SPITTAL: He has a high-average IQ and very low performance levels. But I found out that the school's entire approach is whole language. They don't teach phonics systematically—not the way it really needs to be taught for kids like Chase. He was taught to look at the picture, look for "contextual clues." Basically, it's guessing. Last night, we were reading *The Cats of Mrs. Calamari*. There's a sentence about Mrs. Calamari walking down the street with "short, uniformed figures." Chase looked at the picture and said "soldiers." And I said, "Chase, that's not what the book says. Let's read the words in the book." And he said emphatically: "You're supposed to look at the pictures to figure out if the pictures could help you read the book. You look for clues in the pictures." And I said, "Well, Chase, someday there aren't going to *be* any pictures, and you need to learn how to read the words." And so we walked through "sh, o, r, t, uniformed figures." And he didn't guess anymore last night. But that was my first real confrontation with him on guessing because it's not going to help him when there are no pictures.

Q: Where do you go from here?

SPITTAL: I've hired an Orton-Gillingham tutor. She works with Chase twice a week.

Q: Is it a financial hardship to come up with the $225 a month for tutoring?

SPITTAL: Chase's dad and I are going to split the cost. We'd like to get the school to pay for it, although I don't really think that will happen. But I understand from what I've read that the school is supposed to provide him with a teacher who can teach him the way he needs to learn. That's part of a free-and-appropriate education under IDEA. If *they* can't teach him because their teachers aren't trained to, then they are supposed to find somebody who can. I know that Chase has rights, and they need to teach him in a way that he can understand it.

Q: What do you think would have happened to Chase if you hadn't been such a strong advocate for him?

SPITTAL: He absolutely would have fallen through the cracks, just like so many other kids are falling through the cracks because there is no guidance out there for parents, even parents who are very concerned about their child's reading level.

"THE SHAME OVERSHADOWS YOUR LIFE"

The contemporary West Hills home where Debra Brooks lives with her banker husband and her three teenage kids gives only one visible clue to the learning disability that has dogged her life: the fridge. Most families stick notes on their refrigerator door with Scotch tape or magnets. But Brooks, whose dyslexia and attention disorder play havoc with her efforts to organize her life, has abandoned paper notes for a door that's 100-percent scrawl-able. The slate-fronted refrigerator serves as a chalkboard where she can jot down appointments, keep track of her children's activities, and make lists of groceries to buy. "It's a dyslexic's dream," the forty-eight-year-old Portlander says of the double-duty appliance.

The refrigerator-cum-day planner is just one of the countless strategies Brooks has devised over the years to cope with her disability at home, in school, and in her twenty-year career as a social worker and clinical therapist. Her serene suburban life, led in a house full of color, art, and comfortable good taste, has a dark subtext of pain and struggle. "There's a sense of shame that accompanies the syndrome of dyslexia," she says. "The shame overshadows your whole life."

Sitting in her sunny kitchen, her hands wrapped around a mug of hot coffee, Brooks describes the confusion she felt as a child when she faltered badly in school. Her deep-set green eyes well up with remembered grief as she tells the story of the little girl, the daughter of prominent rabbi Murray Saltzman, who felt herself shrinking away under her parents' anger and disapproval. She confesses to seeking out smart men when she got to college, leaning on them to get her through her bachelor's degree in social work from the University

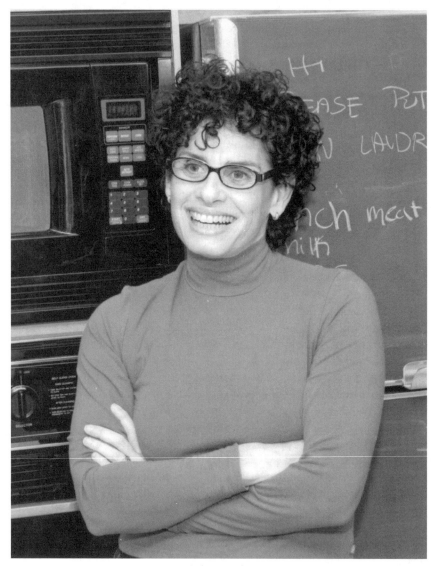

Debra Brooks

of Cincinnati and, eventually, an MSW from Columbia University. She talks about always cultivating a "buddy" in the workplace—someone she could rely on to help manage the paperwork and administrative details that are, for dyslexics, like circling sharks, always waiting to take you down. "It was detrimental, needing somebody to help me learn and doing whatever it took to get that person to help me, even if it meant compromising myself," she says with regret in her voice.

Sick of the struggle to hide her disability, tired of trying to outswim the sharks, Brooks recently has turned to face her inner adversary. After butting heads for years with an abusive boss at one of the Northwest's largest health-care providers, she has set out on her own to help other learning-disabled workers by offering trainings to employers about dyslexia in the workplace. She has also turned her hand to writing, recently publishing several Internet articles—"Dyslexia in the Workplace" (*Dyslexia Online Magazine*, May 2004) and "Talk to Me, Radio Man" (www.DiversityWorld.com, November 2004).

"I've finally decided to stop trying to fight it," Brooks says. "Forty-eight years is a long time fighting. It takes so much energy to hide."

Q: When did you realize that you were different from other children?

BROOKS: I first noticed that there was something odd about me when I was in kindergarten and I couldn't tie my shoelaces like the other kids. I can remember as clear as day sitting on the floor and I couldn't grab hold of the string and make the first loop. I felt *bad*. I felt clumsy, like I was all-thumbs. I remember turning around so no one would see that my shoes were untied—and not telling my mom. That was the beginning of the hiding. A child not being able to tell their parents what they're experiencing, or not being believed when they *do* tell, basically lets the child know that they don't exist—that what's inside of them is not there. You feel invisible at times, and invalidated. I had a brother who was eighteen months younger and a quick learner, and I saw how pleased my parents were with his ability to read and his coordination. So I got littler and littler. And I would always tell people, "I'm the oldest!"

Q: As you moved on in school, how did you feel about struggling to learn?

BROOKS: We went to this fancy, very sophisticated school system in Chappaqua, New York, where everything was the latest and top-of-the-line. I was in second grade and couldn't read, and it was always this feeling of blurriness and fumbliness—nothing was ever clear, everything was messy and blurry and I didn't understand it. I couldn't do it. I couldn't write inside the lines. I had the hardest time holding the pencil and not pressing too hard. I always had blisters from holding onto the pencil so tight. I was trying *so hard*. It felt like if I could just hold onto the pencil a little bit harder, I could do it. My parents got me glasses— glasses with blue frames—but I still couldn't read.

Q: Were you getting support, emotionally and educationally, at home?

BROOKS: In the home, I was starting to feel less and less able to do *any-thing*. It felt like I was just the girl on the side with this brilliant brother. I remember these sessions at night with the homework. My mom was a teacher, and she thought I wasn't paying attention. So she would push my head into the book and say, "*Look* at it!" It was terrible. And my dad would scream at her, saying, "She *is* looking at it!" But then *he* would scream at me.

Q: Your father was quite an accomplished man, wasn't he?

BROOKS: My dad's a first-generation American, a Reform rabbi whose father and mother escaped from persecution in Russia in the early 1900s. He was appointed to the U.S. Commission on Civil Rights in the mid '70s. And he had a TV show, *Focus on Faith*. Everybody went to him for guidance. He was an amazing human being. But in our family, to feel loved, to feel accepted, you had to be able to think fast, to read and write like a scholar. I didn't fit, and I felt stupid and guilty and ashamed almost all of the time.

Q: When were you diagnosed with dyslexia?

BROOKS: Around fourth grade—about 1965. By that time, I was feeling pretty bad about myself—*really* bad—on all different levels. My parents saw it. You can tell when a kid doesn't feel good about herself. The school counselor told them I should see a psychologist, but my parents wouldn't take me. They fought it. They didn't want me to feel there was anything wrong with me. It was very strong denial. Their whole focus was, "You just need to try harder." They *did* get me some help with reading. I would sit down with this lady after school—my parents paid for that—and she would do reading lessons with me—phonetics and that kind of thing. She was a very gentle person, never criticized me. I remember starting to feel like I could breathe a little bit. I still had a horrible time spelling—even to this day I can't spell.

Q: You eventually graduated from high school and went to college.

BROOKS: Yes. When I got to the University of Cincinnati, I just took off. I made the dean's list the first semester. But when I went to the University of Pennsylvania for graduate school, I flunked Introduction to Social Work my first quarter. I had to go to the dean's office. As a last-ditch effort, I blurted out the shameful thing that I was always hiding: "I'm dyslexic." I was thinking, "It doesn't matter anyway. They want me to get out of there because I'm no good." Well, they lit up. "Why didn't you tell us?" they asked. "We have funds for you. We'll get you a tutor. Meet with your professor and figure out a different way to test. We'll make accommodations—don't you know the law?" This was about

1980. I took the test over again, orally this time, and got an A. I transferred to Columbia University the next year and got my master's.

Q: How did your dyslexia affect your professional life?

BROOKS: My strength is field work. I've organized career counseling in a residential program for pregnant teens through the Salvation Army and worked with abused foster children through Catholic Charities. I've provided day treatment for schizophrenics in New York City. But I'm not good with paperwork. My most recent boss would get very irritated because I'm not detailed enough. One time, he wouldn't let me go to a conference with everybody else in the department because he said I learn too slowly. I wasn't allowed to make any spelling mistakes. The worst thing you can do to a person with a learning disability is to tell them that they have to spell everything right. It's so ironic, because on the Christmas card he wrote me, he spelled my name wrong.

Q: Why did you decide to start your own business consulting with employers about learning disabled workers?

BROOKS: I wanted to somehow move beyond the pain of this whole experience. All the pain that had built up over the years flooded in again during the conflict with my boss. It made me physically ill. I lost twenty pounds. In the end, I couldn't go to work anymore. I decided to do trainings for employers on how to recognize invisible disabilities, like dyslexia and ADD, and how to have conversations with employees about making accommodations *before* anybody starts calling the EEOC (Equal Employment Opportunity Commission) or attorneys—*way* before.

"WE HAD TO SUE THE SCHOOL"

As is true for many activists in the field of reading disability, Cathy Wyrick's original motivation was primal: the fierce, uncompromising need to nurture and protect her child. When her daughter Edie was just one year old, her husband Bob, then an investigative reporter in Washington, D.C., for *Newsday*, suffered a disabling stroke that left Wyrick to shoulder much of the parenting alone—a challenge that was compounded when Edie turned out to have a learning disability. Wyrick's first tentative steps into the arcane and often acerbic realm of special education on behalf of her little girl led, over the span of two decades, to her current role as executive director of the Blosser Center for Dyslexia Resources, a fledgling nonprofit in Portland, Oregon.

In 1999, Wyrick spearheaded a major challenge to high-stakes testing in a landmark lawsuit called *Advocates for Special Kids* vs. *The State of Oregon*.

Wyrick's team of lawyers argued that if the state was going to require students to pass its Certificate of Initial Mastery for high school graduation—as was the plan at that time—it must provide appropriate accommodations for all kids with documented disabilities. So, for example, a glitch in brain wiring makes spelling nearly impossible for most dyslexics to master, and poses a lifelong challenge. Eighth-grader Edie Wyrick, whose severe dyslexia rendered her a disabled speller, should therefore be allowed to use a computer with a spell-checker for the writing portion of the test. Here's an analogy: Just as it would be illegal under federal law to require a blind student to read the test without a Braille translation, so would it be illegal to require a disabled speller to write an essay without a spell-checker—especially, as was the case in Oregon, when scores on spelling (which isn't taught after sixth grade) were double-weighted. As a result of the suit, Oregon schools agreed to offer alternate tests for kids whose performance is hampered by learning disabilities.

Wyrick has been relentless, not only in her advocacy for LD kids but also in her search for understanding the tangled roots—biological, political, and cultural—that feed the problem. Drawing on her early training as a journalist, she has shown the doggedness of an intrepid reporter in digging for solutions. After earning a master's degree in special ed, she launched the Blosser Center in 2001 with her mentor Dorothy Blosser Whitehead. Yet the primal passion that got her started continues to resonate in her words as she tells her story—a story that starts with the simple love of a mother for her little girl.

Q: When did your daughter Edie's reading problems first show up?

WYRICK: The neighborhood Montessori preschool she was going to in Washington, D.C., was doing some reading activities and she wasn't picking it up. Then she went to an all-day kindergarten, and Edie really started resisting at that point. She was spending her time under the desk or in her cubby. The teacher complained that Edie wouldn't come in from the playground—that she was irritating other kids and that she was just generally a "bad" kid. We had a very nasty discussion. The teacher accused her of ruining her class.

Q: What did you do then?

WYRICK: I called a psychologist who said we'd better have Edie tested. By that point, she was in first grade. The psychologist called after the first three hours of testing and said, "Well, you'd better start looking for a school because this child is dyslexic—it's an open-and-shut case." She finished the private testing and then the school district wanted to do their own testing, but of course, because of the backup it would be three months before they would get to it. Meanwhile, Edie would come home every day, crying and saying, "Why can my friend read and I can't? What's the matter with me?"

Q: So what was the final straw?

WYRICK: We had started looking for private schools, but first you have to fight with the school district because they don't *want* you to go looking for schools. Things had gotten so bad that I couldn't bear to leave her there all day, so I had started taking her home at lunchtime. One day, I came to pick her up and she wasn't in her classroom. One little girl said she'd seen Edie walk away during recess. To get to our apartment from her school, which is near the Washington Cathedral, you had to cross Connecticut Avenue—a six-lane boulevard. I was fighting panic, trying to stay calm, trying to think of where she might go. The school counselor jumped in her car and went one way, and I went the other way. When the counselor found her, she was two blocks away from Connecticut Avenue sitting under a tree. I said to her, "Gee, you must be feeling pretty bad to walk away by yourself." She said, "No, Mom, I feel pretty good because I'm not at school anymore."

Q: How did the school respond to the incident?

WYRICK: The incident speeded up the assessment process. After a series of tests they gave Edie the very next day, they said, "Well, no question—Edie is dyslexic." After some legal action—we had to sue the school to get an outside placement—Edie went to Kingsbury Day School, which is a private school for kids with learning disabilities.

Q: What was Edie like at home when she wasn't worried about her reading?

WYRICK: Edie had always been an active child—real physical. She was a teeny-tiny little thing and she liked to climb and slide and do roly-poly kinds of games. She liked dress-up, drama, dancing. One day she was watching our family cat, and she said, "Mom, want to see how Connie White walks?" And she did this amazing imitation, sort of rolling her shoulders in a fluid, feline way.

Q: What about your reading habits as a family?

WYRICK: I read many, many books to her. We started out with the 1-2-3 kind of books. And my husband and I read all the time, so she saw plenty of people reading. She was always high verbal.

Q: What was going through your mind and your heart as you watched Edie struggle?

WYRICK: It's extremely frightening, especially when you have a teacher who's telling you that your child is making her life miserable. There was no sympathy from the school, no understanding. At the public school in Washington, D.C., the principal and teachers didn't want to know about

Edie's disability. They figured it was all my fault. They would imply that there must be something wrong at home. This kindergarten teacher actually told me flat-out that I wasn't disciplining Edie enough, and that if I would only exert more discipline—by that she meant physical punishment—then she would do her work on time. She saw Edie's behavior as being balky and irritating on purpose. As a parent, you don't know where to go.

Q: Besides hiring a private tutor and sending Edie to private schools, what other supports did you provide to Edie during her school years?

WYRICK: She got into clay animation through a community-based enrichment program for kids. She was always interested in motion; in animation, you have to break movements down into little pieces and to think sequentially. It really helped her to focus on sequencing, which so many dyslexics struggle with. She also went to a summer camp where they do shortened versions of famous plays, including works by Shakespeare. Reading Shakespeare in high school English classes was no problem for her.

Q: Your story is the story of an educated mother who was in there advocating every day of the week for her child and who knew how to find resources and how to hire lawyers. But most kids don't have this level of informed parental support.

WYRICK: That's exactly right, and those kids don't get anything. That's the crime. When I was teaching tutors at Chief Joseph Elementary School, a nice little school in a working-class neighborhood, one of the children was this little African American guy, a fifth-grader. On his pre-test, he was pretty much a nonreader. But after our tutor worked with him for seven months, he was almost at grade level. I felt real happy. As I left the school building at the end of the year, his teacher said, "Oh, he's done so well. We were sure he was retarded." How could *anybody* think this child was retarded? He had a good vocabulary, he was smart and cute and talkative. I was really depressed as I drove across town to Oregon Episcopal School, where I was sitting in on an IEP meeting for a boy I was going to start tutoring. Well, he had a whole team of teachers there, a $5,000 private evaluation—all this kind of stuff—and it was like night and day. That's why I'm working to build the nonprofit Blosser Center, to teach more teachers how to work with struggling readers so kids like the little guy at Chief Joseph can have the benefit of tutoring. It should be available to everyone.

Q: So in 1994 you enrolled in a master's program in special ed with the idea of working with LD kids like Edie.

WYRICK: Yes, but most of the special ed programs at colleges of education nationwide are focused on children with severe physical or mental disabilities. There was a chapter on mental retardation, a chapter on learning disabilities, chapters on autism, physical disability, blindness and deafness, and they were all given equal weight—even though learning disabilities are, proportionally, vastly more prevalent among the disabled population.

Q: Did you go to work in the school district?

WYRICK: Are you ready for another story from hell? I was doing student teaching in a ninth-grade English class. Every kid in this group of twenty-five had an IEP for learning disabilities. They were all dyslexic. The teacher spent every day reminding them that they were stupid, they were lazy, they were never going to go to college, and she didn't even know why they were there. This horrible woman would walk into the room and the students would just kind of sink down. One night there was a movie on TV with Kirk Douglas or Lloyd Bridges, or one of these big stars, about a dyslexic man who discovers his dyslexia and learns how to read. It was a big deal, a Hallmark Hall of Fame production. All these kids had seen it, and they were sitting up straight, all enthusiastic, wanting to talk about it. The teacher says, "Yeah, I saw that," and one of the kids said, "Kirk Douglas, he's dyslexic, too." She said, "Well, it couldn't possibly be because he's smart and he wrote a book. So he can't be dyslexic." All these kids just sank back down into oblivion again.

Q: Do the kids seem bored during a forty-five-minute lesson on sounds and blending?

WYRICK: Sometimes. But the important question is, is this therapeutic? It's a medical model. It's more like physical therapy than anything else. It's not necessarily fun. But if, after a couple of months, the child realizes she can do these things that she could never do before, then she has bought into it. She wants to get onto the next step. A lot of educators criticize this approach as being boring, but for kids who find reading to be very mysterious, they finally get a handle on it.

Q: Do you think this approach is valuable not only for dyslexic kids, but for kids who are having trouble reading for other reasons—because, perhaps, they didn't have much literacy background in their home?

WYRICK: The National Institutes of Health research shows that there's a continuum of reading ability and disability. It's just like singing: Some people are divas and some people can't carry a tune. And, like singing, reading has the same relationship to intelligence: none. Some kids, if you put a book in front of them at age four, they can read. Other kids struggle terribly. And there's this whole continuum in between. It's a matter of how much phonics somebody needs. Some people just need a little bit to kind of clue them in to the system. Other people need the "physical therapy" level.

Q: Many educators don't believe there is such a thing as dyslexia.

WYRICK: Right. They think these kids are just lazy and stupid.

Q: Why would you not believe in dyslexia when there's scientific evidence coming from places like Yale?

WYRICK: I've had people say, "Well, you can make science say whatever you want." It also has to do with the definition of intelligence. People want to believe that reading and intelligence are the same thing. They want to believe that spelling and intelligence are the same thing. They can't get over that hump, this stubborn belief that if you can't do those simple things—read, spell—then you must not be smart.

Q: Why is phonics linked in many people's minds with the conservative cultural agenda?

WYRICK: Some conservative groups have glommed onto phonics because they like things that seem old-fashioned—you know, the old McGuffey's Readers. They think of those old approaches as reflecting enduring moral values. But why anybody else would think that phonics is somehow "conservative" is bizarre to me. The scientists who are investigating reading instruction are, for the most part, left-wing Democrats. I've gone to conferences where researchers and scholars say they're amazed that people assume their politics are of a certain type. E. D. Hirsch, who developed the Core Knowledge curriculum, gets all kinds of grief. It's a wonderful program—direct instruction in the classics, in all these things you need to know to be successful at top-flight colleges. He's a left-wing Democrat with a dyslexic son. There's no reason why reading should be a political issue at all. Reading isn't going to get fixed unless it becomes nonpolitical.

Q: Does Edie's story have a good ending?

WYRICK: Edie's story is a good story now, but it could have been not good at all. She's starting her junior year at the University of Oregon. She's got a B average, and she's gotten A's on philosophy papers. She still can't spell, but she can read really well. She can read any word you put in front of her. And she's not hiding under the table anymore.

THE STORY OF EDIE

What career might a college woman majoring in dance and philosophy envision for herself? Reptile breeding doesn't immediately pop to mind. But Edie

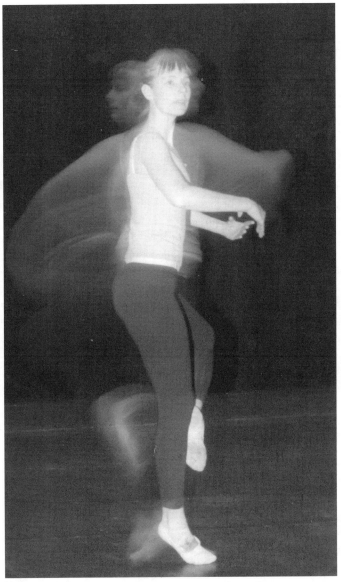

Edie Wyrick

Wyrick thinks the two leopard geckos she and her boyfriend recently purchased as pets are "awesome," and that launching a business raising and selling snakes, lizards, turtles, and other scaly, cold-blooded creatures would be great. "I've always been a reptile girl," says the University of Oregon junior, whose given name is Edith. "First it was dinosaurs, then it was dragons. When I was five, I wanted to be a paleontologist. When I was in fifth grade, I read a lot of fantasy dragon books."

The fact that she *could* read those reptilian fantasies was, for Edie, not something she took for granted. As she talks with us in the university library, dressed in a frayed cotton T-shirt and a pair of faded, floppy pants, she recalls her childhood reading struggles a little reluctantly. With some gentle prodding, snippets of those early years surface in her mind: hiding under desks and in closets to escape the pressures of school. Slipping away from the schoolyard at recess with an urgent wish to go home. Fighting back—and then getting in trouble—when other kids razzed her. Feeling the panic rise in her throat as her first-grade teacher called on kids to read words chalked on the blackboard. Print for Edie was just a meaningless mishmash, a frustrating blur.

Thanks to a diagnosis of dyslexia at age six (and a tenacious mother), Edie was not only an average reader by middle school, she was an honor student. Her new place to hide was in the pages of fantasy novels roiling with fire-breathing dragons, knights in shining armor, and damsels in distress.

But, as is typical with dyslexia, her spelling remained atrocious. On her eighth-grade state writing test, such misspellings as "wen" for "when" and "tryed" for "tried" cancelled out the high marks she earned for style and content, netting her a failing score. When she got to high school, an English teacher tried to boot her out of the honors class because Edie's first essay was riddled with spelling errors.

Her persistent spelling problems became the catalyst for a class-action lawsuit that Edie's mom Cathy brought against the state of Oregon and the Portland School District in 1999. Edie found herself thrust into the media limelight. Giving press conferences and interviews wasn't a role she relished. Like just about every sixteen-year-old kid, she was by then deeply entangled in the universal adolescent conundrum: how to get your homework done and still have a social life. So it was grudgingly that she gave up time with her friends to advocate for kids who, like her, needed accommodations such as spell checkers to pass statewide exams.

"It was kind of weird for me," she says. "I just saw it as something my mom wanted me to do. It was, 'My mom's going off on this weird crusade—oh my God!' I thought it was more her thing than my thing. Now I realize I was just being an idiot."

The biggest coup of the lawsuit's publicity campaign came when the *Wall Street Journal* called. Edie doesn't remember the interview with *Journal* staff reporter Daniel Golden or the page 1 article titled "Will Academic Standards Suffer if Disabled Students Get a Break?" which ran on January 21, 2000. All her media contacts, she admits, "run together" in her memory now.

Edie has long since traded her dragon fantasy novels for the works of the great philosophers, joining the centuries-old quest to understand the human condition. "I like how instead of taking a conclusion and seeing where it leads, philosophy really examines *all* conclusions," Edie says. "And it asks 'Why?' all the time, and 'How can we make things better?' It helps me get grounded in what's actually good. I see so many things that are poorly managed and poorly run, poorly conceived, poorly designed. Philosophy goes with my wanting to get to the bottom of something and fix it. The other thing I like about philosophy is that they always grade on content. So if I have some grammatical things and spelling things, they'll write a note but they won't take it off your grade."

In a way, philosophy has given Edie a new place to hide. "It takes me out of this toxic, stupid world and helps me find a good way to function," she says. "This society does nothing for realizing actual human potential. It even discourages it."

Edie's other place to hide is the dance studio. Dance gives a physical balance to the cerebral realm of her philosophy curriculum. Just as philosophy is, for Edie, a vehicle for seeing beyond everyday assumptions, dance is an exploration of alternatives in aesthetics and the arts. "I like nontraditional music—music that harkens to other art forms, music that has movement in it, that has a swing quality," she says. "I like music that's thoughtful. I like rock—the energy, the raw dissonance. I like things that sound interesting."

"WHAT HAPPENED TO CHUCKY?"

Chuck Arthur is annoyed and embarrassed about the tears that well up, involuntarily, behind his metal-rimmed glasses as he reminisces about his childhood reading troubles. "I was afraid I'd do this," he says, brushing at his eyes irritably. "I wish I weren't doing this."

For most of his adult life, his boyhood sense of shame had been forgotten. So he couldn't have been more surprised when, during a visit to Illinois for his forty-fifth high school reunion, he broke down and wept in his older sister's kitchen. Nothing that has happened in the last half-century—not his successful teaching career, not his graduate degree in special ed, not his in-depth

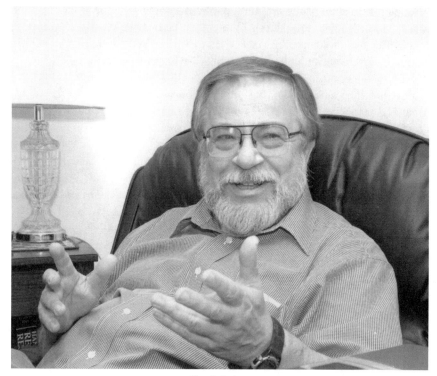

Chuck Arthur

study of the roots of learning disability—had erased the pain of the family secret about the boy who couldn't read.

Arthur didn't consciously choose a career path that led him to teach kids who, just like him, have great difficulty unraveling the secrets of print. Yet, maybe pulled by a subliminal tug from his own buried anguish, he was drawn inexorably toward special ed. From his first experiences with students whose behavior put them on the outs with the mainstream, he grasped the central role of reading failure. Once kids started to read, he found, their behavior improved. Pretty soon, Arthur was absorbing everything he could find about why so many kids struggle with reading and latching on to materials that, despite their vilification in the wider education community, were turning around the lives of children once deemed hopeless.

At age sixty-four, most people are ready to hit the recliner with a stack of novels, or hit the golf course in a pair of loud shorts. But Arthur has launched a whole new phase of his career, opening a K–3 charter school called Arthur Academy in the David Douglas School District. The cluster of modular classrooms out among the taverns, cheap motels, and convenience stores along Division Street in Portland's blue-collar East County has done astounding work with a diverse population of kids, many from tough circumstances, including immigrants from Mexico and Russia. In 2004, the second year of the school's operation, the kindergarten class—kids with names like Karma and Angel, Mahkayla and Omri, Baylee and Chance—had an average score in the 89th percentile on an end-of-year national reading test—up from the 36th percentile at the start of the year. Half of them reached the 99th percentile.

Inevitably, the phonics-based academy has raised some hackles. An article in the September 18, 2004, issue of *The Oregonian* tells about a few prickly moments when, after the Portland School Board voted to approve an Arthur charter in the city's main district, one member appended the discussion with a "word of caution" about his methods. "He started to get almost like a bull that was in a pen snorting and kicking the ground, ready to charge," Rob Kremer, the director of the Oregon Public Charter School Service Center, told *Oregonian* reporter Tracy Jan. "I had to catch his eye and say, 'Now Chuck, we've won. This is her last parting shot. It doesn't matter. Settle down.'"

Arthur, professorial in his gray beard and rumpled blue shirt, just can't help but bristle a little at the criticism. But mostly, he responds to the naysayers with a shrug and a simple retort that's hard to argue with: "It works."

Confident in his command of the research and his lifetime of experience, he's been busy extending his academy into neighboring communities, opening two new schools in 2004 and two more in 2005. The small, plastic reader board that welcomes visitors to every Arthur Academy telegraphs the founder's mission in two words: "Everybody reads."

Q: Talk about your own childhood experiences with struggling to read.

ARTHUR: I grew up in rural Maine. My folks were educated, but I was one of the worst readers in the class. Then we moved down to the Boston area where I went to a middle-class, suburban school, but I still wasn't learning how to read. My mother used to worry like crazy. She'd take every opportunity to try to help Chucky learn how to read. When we'd go to church, we'd sing hymns and she'd move her finger under every word. I remember feeling very, very puzzled about why I couldn't read because all my friends could read. I felt very defeated, hopeless. In the third grade I got two F's. My teacher told my mother—this is the story that has been passed around our family—"Chucky's going to be a late bloomer."

Q: Did anyone try to diagnose the problem?

ARTHUR: This was in the late '40s. Nobody knew anything about dyslexia in those days. I thought I wasn't smart, and I think that assumption
was even subtly communicated to me in my family. My younger sister
had learning problems, too, but my older sister was smart, and then
along comes my younger brother and outsmarts us all. "Look how
Bobby can read!" The implication was, "What happened to Chucky?"

Q: But you eventually got to college.

ARTHUR: Yes, but when I took these tests to get into college, I did very
badly. The woman who reviewed the test scores met with me to go over
the results. I vividly remember sitting in the library office and her saying, "You're not college material." I remember thinking, "Yes, I am!" I
knew I had to go to college.

Q: What did you do?

ARTHUR: In those days, it was easier to get into state schools. I had
played trombone in the band, and I decided to be a music major at the
hometown college. I was thinking I would become a band director, so I
wouldn't have to take many academic classes. I put off all the heavy-
duty classes. I failed the first-semester of English, but luckily I had taken
enough music classes to maintain a passing average. The worst classes
were history because I couldn't do the volume of reading. I could understand what I read, but I couldn't keep up, although I liked history a lot.
Finally, the class I was putting off the most was philosophy. Oh, wow,
philosophy! As it turns out, that doesn't require a *lot* of reading; it
requires *careful* reading and thought. Well, I got the only A in the class.
By then I knew I wasn't dumb. I was beginning to change my view of
myself. I found out that although I was a slow reader, I could comprehend and deal with ideas and information once I read the material.

Q: How and why did you get into teaching?

ARTHUR: After graduate school, I took a job teaching fifth grade. I
thought teaching was going to be temporary until I found something
more exciting, but I got hooked. Before I started, I didn't even know
there was such a thing as special education. I eventually got a job in
Boston teaching kids with behavior problems—all different varieties
under the heading of "behavior disorder." The commonality was that
almost none of them could read—they were older kids reading at the
second-grade level. Behavior-problem kids almost always have learning
problems, and I quickly learned that it's the learning problems you can
most likely attack. If you can get to the learning problems, you'll have
a ton of effect on the behavior. All of a sudden, their emotional state at
school changed, and the psychologist who wanted to psychoanalyze
these kids was amazed at their improved behavior.

Q: What teaching strategies were you using?

ARTHUR: I attended a Troubled Child Conference at the University of Oregon, and I had heard Zig Engelmann talk about the DISTAR program. And I thought, "Yeah, that's the one that's been researched." I was trying to find better tools. So I bought the Corrective Reading curriculum. And it worked with these kids. I was finding out that if you did systematic instruction with the alphabetic system that was phonetically controlled, you could be very successful. I tried using high-interest stuff, but that wasn't enough because there were always a lot of words in the high-interest material that they couldn't read. The rule was, I had to give them things they could do.

Q: How much improvement did the students achieve in their reading skills?

ARTHUR: Two grade levels a year. Then I went to the wealthy community of Winchester, Massachusetts, to work with a group of junior high kids who were reading at second- and third-grade levels. They had normal intelligence, and they were nice little kids. So why weren't they learning? The school didn't know what to do with these misfits in this rich community. They had just slipped by.

Q: What happened when they started getting direct instruction?

ARTHUR: Once again, we were able to bring them up two grade levels each year.

Q: Describe your approach to reading instruction at Arthur Academy.

ARTHUR: We teach reading in very careful pieces. Our approach is based on one axiom: Every lesson that we present to the kids, they're all able to do. Our goal is to make sure every lesson here is successful—*every* lesson. If a kid isn't successful by the end of the lesson, it's not the right lesson for them or they're in the wrong group. Of course, you could always be successful if you kept it easy all the time, but you also have to make sure that each lesson leads to accelerated progress. That's quite a trick to pull off.

Q: Would you call it a mastery-learning approach?

ARTHUR: Yeah. Each lesson has to be mastered; otherwise, the child isn't ready to move on. You think about what that means to the kids. They always know that when we call on them, we're going to ask them something they can do. They become very confidant in themselves—"Hey, I'm pretty smart." Each lesson evolves through a mixture of the old with just a little bit of new.

Q: So success is the biggest motivator for kids?

ARTHUR: Yes. But they have to experience the teacher saying, over a period of time, "Oh, you do that quite well." The child goes, "Yeah, that felt pretty good." I can remember convincing even older kids. I'd say,

"I will show you how to read, and you're going to be successful right from the beginning." They'd laugh, act indifferent—"Ha, ha, ha, so what?" That was their attitude. These were kids who were in eighth grade and still reading at a second-grade level. I had to hook them into it, but once you get them hooked, they will come to you every day demanding, "Come on, let's do it."

Q: So it would be impossible for a kid to fall between the cracks in this type of program. There's not going to be some kid in second grade who you suddenly realize can't read?

ARTHUR: Holy mackerel, no.

Q: There's an attitude among many teachers that phonics is a product of the far-right religious community. When you try to talk to a lot of teachers, you can't get past that.

ARTHUR: Yes, I taught a continuing education class at Portland State University in how to strengthen reading skills with phonics. Some of the young teachers in there were shocked to find out that I was a member of the Democratic Party. They couldn't believe it. They were convinced that I was a Republican activist—some right-winger. I'm a liberal Democrat. For some odd reason, whole-language people seem to be liberals. We liberals are suckers for a romantic view of childhood. And when it comes to testing, liberals have been really opposed. They've been misinformed on what testing is all about. You know, we've got some real prejudices on that whole political scene.

"IT'S NEVER BORING!"

We were sitting in the tiny Portland office of Arthur Academy, talking with Chuck Arthur about the skills-based approach to beginning reading that distinguishes his growing chain of charter schools. "How do you answer the critics who say, 'You're doing drill and kill and you're boring the children to death'?" we asked.

"They're wrong," he argued vehemently. "They only think that because they haven't come in to see for themselves. All you have to do is come in and take a look. These are not bored kids."

We pressed the issue. "So maybe it's actually the *teachers* who get bored doing this type of instruction." At that moment, the quick footsteps we could hear coming down the hallway suddenly stopped, and a voice called out emphatically from behind the portable screen, "It's *never* boring!" Arthur looked amused. "Come on in, Alison," he encouraged, then to us, "Alison is a first-grade teacher."

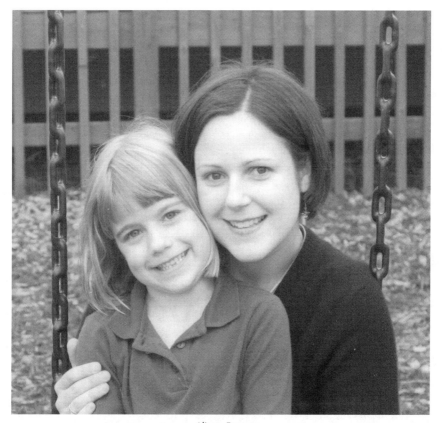

Alison Post

A thirty-something woman with dark hair and an earnest face came around the divider and looked at us, a flash of defiance in her eyes. She didn't know who we were or why we were questioning the techniques that she and the other teachers use at their little charter school, but she wanted to set us straight. "I *love* these programs," she said. "I never get bored with them."

We coaxed her into stopping and talking with us for a few minutes.

Q: Why are you so adamant in your support for direct instruction?

ALISON POST: I was trained in direct instruction when I was doing graduate work in special education at the University of Oregon. Last year was my first year teaching, and I was hired to work with LD kids in a big urban district. I took a beating because my methodological philosophies were so loathed in that district.

Q: What happened?

POST: In my interview, my principal to-be asked me what programs I had worked with. I rattled off a list of at least seven or eight programs, all direct instruction. She hired me, so I assumed I would be able to use those programs. But when I got there and told her I had put in an order for Reading Mastery, she said, "Oh, I saw kids doing that once when I was a teacher, and they looked so bored." She canceled my orders. I was forced—well, forced is a strong word—*almost* forced to use Guided Reading, which is not systematic.

Q: Would you describe Guided Reading as a whole-language approach that encourages kids to guess the words from context?

POST: Yes.

Q: Why did you go into special education?

POST: I was a child who struggled. I had a lot of trouble in school.

Q: Why did you choose UO?

POST: I got lucky; going to UO was serendipity. I got trained in what I consider the most research-based type of instruction available. Special-ed kids can make up a full year of progress with these programs.

Q: So how did you happen upon the Arthur Academy?

POST: I was telling one of my colleagues about being so disappointed with the situation. You've been trained as a specialist in special education, and they hire you because of your expertise, but then you have no control over what curriculum to use for your students. So my colleague said, "Do you know Chuck Arthur and the Arthur Academy? They use all direct instruction programs." My pay is a little less at the charter school, but I gained a couple of spoonfuls of sanity.

"THE PROGRAM IS PART
OF THE HEALING PROCESS"

Cindy Stadel can toss off all kinds of statistics about literacy in America. But there's one number that, no matter how many times she recites it, always leaves her feeling stunned. Whenever she tells people that four-fifths of Oregon offenders left high school without finishing, the enormity of the number knocks her back on her heels. "I was dumbfounded when I heard that, and I'm still dumbfounded," she says, sitting in the downtown Portland office she occupies as administrator of the Londer Learning Center, where hundreds of parolees and probationers have earned their GEDs in its ten-year history. The link between crime and illiteracy couldn't be expressed more pointedly, she believes, than it is in that single statistic.

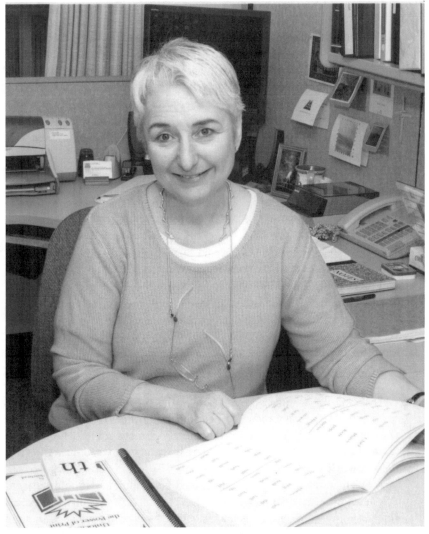

Cindy Stadel

When Stadel was earning her master's degree in communications at New York's Syracuse University thirty-some years ago, her internship with an international literacy nonprofit group became the unintentional launching pad for her career. She was, she admits, a naïve college kid without a shred of awareness about adult literacy issues when she applied at Laubach Literacy International. She couldn't have known then that the "fluky" opportunity, which she figured was just a short-term stint, would lead her into her life's work.

But she got hooked. She saw that literacy, which as the child of a comfortable middle-class family she had taken for granted, was the big missing piece in so many troubled lives. She was disturbed by the irony of an affluent society that guarantees a free education to every child, yet somehow fails to teach and to graduate millions of kids. So she dedicated her life to helping adults get the reading skills and school credentials they missed as children because of learning disabilities, poor instruction, chaotic homes, or—quite often—all three of those factors.

The roughly 600 offenders who come through the center every year often lack even the rudimentary literacy skills needed for basic participation in the economy and the democratic process. Take voting, for instance. On the autumn afternoon we met with Stadel—November 3, the day after the hotly contested 2004 presidential election—the reception area just outside her office was festooned with red, white, and blue streamers. The patriotic decor was left over from a voting workshop held for Londer Center students, most of whom had never cast a ballot before. Seeing the pride with which these first-time voters marked their mail-in ballots is the sort of thing that makes Stadel do what she does.

Even three decades after stumbling into her calling, she still loves to tell the stories of transformation she observes in her work.

Q: Who among your clients comes to mind as a recent triumph?

STADEL: There are just so many stories here—incredible stories. One example is Odis Payton. When his probation officer referred him to the Learning Center in his late thirties, he was a meth addict who couldn't read. When we gave him a reading assessment, his scores were very, very low. He just sat there crying. At his first reading class, he got angry and stormed out, saying, "I don't need no reading!" He told us later, "You know, I tried so many times." Research has said that to have an impact on criminal attitudes and behavior, you need to change thought patterns before you can change behavior. So we got him into a "cog" class—cognitive behavior change—and we had him work on what was he telling himself. Meanwhile, he got glasses and he got new teeth through the Oregon Health Plan. Dental issues are huge for meth addicts. Their teeth begin to decay and their faces literally cave in. Finally, he began engaging in the reading class and started enjoying himself. He even did some acting in a play that one of our teachers directed about the arrest of Susan B. Anthony, the women's-rights crusader.

Q: From your early work in the general area of adult literacy, how did you move toward working specifically with offenders?

STADEL: I took a job teaching at the county jail and realized right away that was where my real passion was. I thought, "Wow, if I want to work with adult nonreaders, where are they? They're in our jails and in our prisons." When I looked at the statistics here in Oregon, I saw that 79 percent of the people in the correction system did not make it in the school system. My God, 79 percent! It's just heartbreaking that the schools aren't working for this population.

Q: What kind of reading skills do your clients have when they first show up here?

STADEL: Today, 65 percent of the people who are coming to us are reading *below* a ninth-grade level.

Q: How has the approach to instruction changed over the past decade?

STADEL: The original goal was to help people get their GED. They needed to have reading skills at a ninth-grade level or above to be successful. We did well with those people. We had a harder time working with the people who were reading at the lower-grade ranges. We were turning over the really hard-to-serve people to our volunteers. The most effective volunteer we had was a woman who was using Orton-Gillingham multisensory techniques, one-to-one. Her students slowly but surely made progress. Then the U.S. Department of Education launched a study looking at the effectiveness of phonics-based programs—decoding—in adult literacy settings. I volunteered the center to join the study, and we adopted the Wilson Reading System, which is another multisensory curriculum that teaches sound-symbol relationships directly and systematically. I then hired another instructor who was using O-G and, once again, she began having success. So we did staff training in both Wilson and Orton-Gillingham. The program now has a lot of integrity for those lower-skilled people.

Q: So some clients are coming in with essentially zero reading skills?

STADEL: Oh, yes. About 15 percent of our clients come in reading at or below a fifth-grade level. We hear them talking about their difficulties in school and how they fell farther and farther behind. At least 85 percent of the people we work with are substance abusers, and many of them started using drugs or alcohol when they began failing in school. It's all tied together. This program is part of the healing process. It provides closure to that unsuccessful secondary-school experience.

Q: Teaching adults to read is a different process than teaching little kids, isn't it?

STADEL: For adults, there's a real need to tie instruction to what they're doing in their daily lives—being able to get a driver's license, to vote, shop, fill out the monthly report we require here at probation. Those very practical, functional-literacy skills are critical. So we've tried to put those two pieces together—to blend the basic-skills instruction with the applied skills. We participate very actively in the county library's Everybody Reads project, where students and reading groups throughout the community all read and discuss a certain novel. Wow! Talk about moving.

Q: Why was it moving?

STADEL: The first book we read was *A Lesson before Dying* by Ernest Gaines. It's a story about a man who can't read and is finally learning to read in jail, but then is executed for a crime he didn't commit. We had people crying. The Reading One students had difficulty reading the book on their own, so we played it for them on audiotape and they followed along. Odis participated in Everybody Reads, and in a letter to the library thanking them for sponsoring the program, he wrote, "What I liked most about *A Lesson before Dying* is it's real to the heart."

Q: Is the investment in terms of taxpayer dollars worth it?

STADEL: We wouldn't have survived as long as we have if there wasn't a payoff. We've had a number of studies that tell us it's working. A county study found that people who had put in at least twenty hours at the center had fewer technical violations on probation and parole, fewer absconds, and higher employment than people with five hours or less at the center. The impact was statistically significant. More recently, the research and evaluation unit of the county's Department of Community Justice looked at 343 offenders who had participated in the center between 1995 and 2001. They found that two-thirds of the center participants made gains of at least one year's growth in reading and/or math, or passed a GED test. Arrests were down significantly during the two-year period following participation in the program. The impact is very positive.

"I'M STARTING TO CATCH ON, CATCH ON, CATCH ON"

For little "Tony," learning to read was like trying to grab a slippery fish in a murky pond. Whatever meanings his schoolbooks contained were darting shadows, always eluding his grasp. When, as a twenty-year-old man, he enrolled in the Londer Learning Center after serving two months in jail after an altercation with his girlfriend, Tony was nearly illiterate. A test revealed that the probationer had a reading level of about second grade.

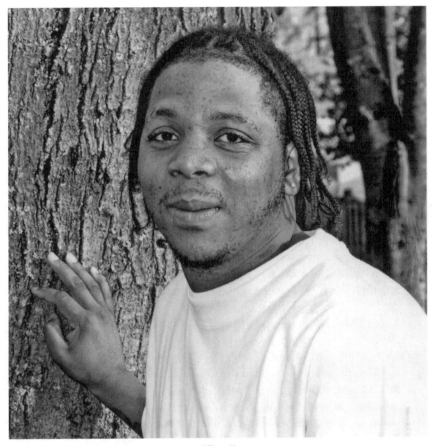

"Tony"

But after only a few hours of intensive tutoring at the center, he began to see the random print around him coalesce into meaningful messages. The marks on street signs and billboards were suddenly more than just inscrutable scrawls. The headlines on newspapers made sense and drew him in. At restaurants, he could read the menu instead of faking it to save face in front of his date. Best of all, when his children toddled over and climbed onto his lap with a storybook in their hands, he didn't have to say, "Not now, honey—I'm too busy to read to you."

The breakthrough Tony has made under the determined tutelage of the center's administrator Cindy Stadel hasn't transformed his life completely. Another fight with the mother of one of his three kids recently landed him behind bars for a second time. He's off supervision now and working part-time as a janitor cleaning offices in the high-rises of downtown Portland.

It's clear that Tony's difficult school years, which ended when he was booted out of an alternative program at fourteen or fifteen, still bother him. But his delight in finally cracking the alphabetic code is obvious, too. Wearing a green, quilted jacket and a white "doo-rag" over the rows of tiny braids in his glossy black hair, Tony talks with animation about getting effective reading lessons at last. Charming and articulate as he speaks candidly in the African American dialect of his blue-collar neighborhood, he doesn't comment on the irony of finally getting the help he needed only after becoming caught up in the justice system. He holds little bitterness toward a school system that didn't work for him. He's focused now on making sure his own kids master the reading skills that for him always seemed beyond his reach.

Q: What are your earliest memories of trying to read in school?

TONY: I went to preschool and I attended elementary school every day, but it seemed like my mind wouldn't pay attention to reading. It'll pay attention to everything else, but it won't pay attention to reading. To this day, it's really hard to read. But I mean, I came kind of far from where I used to be. So I'm proud of myself for that.

Q: What are you learning?

TONY: Well, Cindy don't just say, "OK, see if you can read it." She explains to you how to sound the word out, to make you understand how to read. She shows you the basics of reading. Now I'm starting to catch on, catch on, and catch on. Since I've been working with her, I can drive down the street and read a word like that [he snaps his fingers] because I know how to sound it out. Before, I'd be stuck on that word for days. They could pay me a million dollars, and I wouldn't know how to say that word.

Q: What are some of the drawbacks of being a nonreader?

TONY: One bad thing about not being able to read is going to fill out your own applications and stuff like that. And it's kind of hard for me to go to a restaurant and try to order off the menu. I mean, I might want to go to a restaurant where they don't have picture food. I might be out on a date and don't want to tell this woman, "Hey, can you read this to me because I can't read?" You know, it's like real embarrassing. It hurts, you know, it hurts. Another bad thing is not being able to read a story-book. I've got three beautiful kids. My son is four, his name's Ray Quan. My daughter's name is Sierra, and she's three. My other one is Tony Jr., and he's nine months. Ray Quan would come up to me, or Sierra would come up to me and say, "Daddy, can you read to me?" And I feel like, if I would never had Cindy, I would have never been able to even read a sentence of those books to my children.

Q: You said Cindy shows you how to sound out the word and figure it out. Didn't your teachers do that when you were in first or second grade?

TONY: No. I never had a teacher like Cindy where they'd get down to the bottom—show you how to do the basic things in reading instead of, like I said, just putting the book in front of you. She breaks the words down. She separates them so they're small words and you just blend them together.

Q: The syllables?

TONY: Yeah, syllables. The main thing that's been really, really clicking into my mind and catching on is segmenting the words—pulling them apart and pushing them together, sounding them out, little piece by little piece. You just blend the syllables together and the word will automatically just state itself.

Q: Did your brothers and sisters have trouble with reading?

TONY: I'm the only one in the family that had a problem like this. My brother, he graduated from high school, straight-A student, no problems, honor roll, student of the year. And both my sisters got good marks and they could read and write. My mom, she's a strong black woman, you know, she holded three jobs down to take care of all of us. She always was there for us when we needed something. She always was there to teach us about our homework. She used to read to us all the time. She used to be real, real strict on me about this situation and try to help me as much as she can. I used to have a tutor from University of Portland who come to read to me and help me read books.

Q: How long did you stay in school?

TONY: I got kicked out of an alternative school when I was fourteen or fifteen. I was real hyperactive so they wanted me to take Ritalin. My grandma said Ritalin ain't nothing but a drug, like speed, and leads people to other stuff. She didn't want me to take it, so I used to act like I'm taking them and throw them in the garbage can. My advocate, she got fed up and she just told me to leave and don't ever come back.

Q: What kind of grades did you get before you left school?

TONY: Actually, I was getting good grades in everything. I mean, my reading was always "needs improvement," but I was still passing all my classes because I was there on time and know what I was doing. It was just reading class—every time I had reading class, I used to just make up excuses not to read and stuff.

"THE GUY COULDN'T READ A LICK"

From Carrie Swanson's hometown of Echo, it's only a few miles along the winding Umatilla River to Pendleton, famous for Indian blankets and bucking broncos. But each morning when Swanson picks up her portable electronic alarm from the guard at Pendleton's medium-security prison, the sleepy glen of Echo seems about as far away as you can get. After thirteen years as a special-ed teacher for convicts at Eastern Oregon Correctional Institution, Swanson is nonplussed by the steely coils of razor wire glinting on the perimeter of the massive brick complex that once housed mental patients. The daughter of a cowboy and a librarian, Swanson makes good use of both facets of her heritage—the rugged ranch hand and the refined bookworm—in bringing literacy to convicts.

Employed by Blue Mountain Community College as an educational diagnostician, Swanson is under contract to the Department of Corrections (DOC) to identify and guide inmates with learning disabilities. Of the 180 prisoners taking classes at EOCI, she says, about a third are LD.

In the classroom, where she works with groups of twelve inmates in ninety-minute blocks, Swanson's job is not unlike that of any reading teacher. Yet the extreme regimentation of prison life can make even the smallest victories

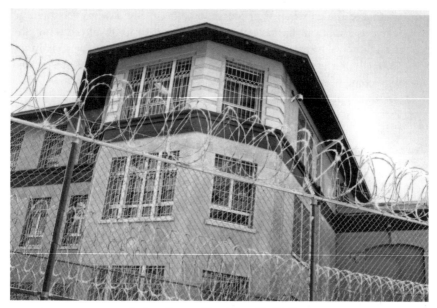

Eastern Oregon Correctional Institution

for literacy hard-won. For instance, she mounted a campaign with prison officials to allow electronic dictionaries for inmates. Five years later, she won. To outsiders unversed in prison culture, it's hard to imagine how a cell-block full of spelling whizzes could be viewed a security threat. It's because, Swanson explains, some inmates use the most innocent, everyday items to cajole or coerce one another. Candy bars can be bargaining chips. Felt-pen ink can wind up in an inmate's arm as a tattoo. Batteries are a highly coveted barter item, apt to cause trouble between weaker and stronger prisoners—so prison rules allow inmates only so many batteries; every alkaline cell must be accounted for.

"The officers come into their personal living space and they literally categorize and check," Swanson says. "So if you paid for a Snickers bar, but not a Hershey bar, and in your possession you have a Hershey bar, then they could assume that you didn't pay for it—that you extorted for that Hershey bar. Therefore, you have an unauthorized item."

Before Swanson took up the cause, an electronic dictionary would put a prisoner over the battery limit. With characteristic doggedness, she dug into the problem.

"I'm a why-not person," she says with a no-big-deal-that's-just-the-way-I-am sort of shrug. "The spell checkers were a big coup. In fact, now they're on the canteen list statewide, and any inmate can buy an electronic dictionary. I have captains signing off on spell checkers. That's pretty neat."

Q: Were you intimidated about working in a prison setting?

SWANSON: I had worked on a fire crew with my husband, so working with men didn't intimidate me. Every one of these 1,300 men here has done something wrong—probably *many* somethings. But it doesn't matter who you are or what you've done: Everybody needs to know how to learn and how to become independent. Oregon law mandates literacy for inmates. So if they read below an eighth-grade level, they're required to go to ninety hours of instruction.

Q: How many learning-disabled inmates were identified as LD before they got here?

SWANSON: There's a difference between the older and younger inmates. The people who've been in the public schools recently—the IDEA kids—more than likely have been tagged already. IDEA (Individuals with Disabilities Education Act) was passed in 1975. That's probably a pretty good marker. They may also have been tagged with a behavior disorder like oppositional-defiance disorder or ADHD. Kids at the facility for delinquent youth fairly commonly have a dual diagnosis of primary, secondary—primary being a behavior disorder, secondary being dyslexia. Thirty of the fifty-four people here who are eligible for special ed have other eligibilities. That could be a physical thing like a seizure disorder, or it could be a mental health issue, or it could be attention deficit. Prior to IDEA, those people were put in a room to make wallets, or they were put in a room with the MR kids [those with intellectual disabililites]. Schools just tended to clump all kids who weren't learning in one place.

Q: Who is the typical inmate who comes to your education program?

SWANSON: I portray them as the lost soul who fell through the cracks. As far as the adults—truck drivers, or whatever they've done for a living—they've maintained gainful employment all their life, but never got a diploma or anything like that. We have a number of guys with high school diplomas who can't read. It used to be, schools didn't know what to do with you, so they just graduated you. To be in the program, they have to have a documented disability.

Q: What triggers an evaluation for learning disabilities here at EOCI?

SWANSON: If they're school age, then we go through IDEA's "Child Find" process. We literally go find those students who are IDEA eligible—the same procedure mandated for public schools—interviewing everyone younger than twenty-two who doesn't have a diploma or has low test scores. We also get referrals from the instructors in the basic-skills program and from corrections staff. And they can self-refer. We have waiting lists, lots of waiting lists, to get into school.

Q: So most of your students felt like failures in school before they got here?

SWANSON: The older the inmate, the more likely you'll run into the, "You mean I'm not stupid after all?" phenomenon. You'll hear a pretty common theme among the men: "This is the first time I've been able to learn."

Q: Do the men talk about what it was like being in public school with a disability?

SWANSON: When I interview them before the assessment session—you know, "What kind of special classes have you been in?"—the older people say, "I was in a class for dummies," or that kind of thing. Most of them come in with little or no understanding of their learning disability, so they have no idea whether they were well served in school. The naiveté of these kids about what they're entitled to in school is pretty huge.

Q: Do they talk about feeling demeaned or inadequate on the outside?

SWANSON: The older people have some sad stories. One guy was in the military, and like a lot of LD people, directionality was a big problem for him. He couldn't do left, right, left, right to save his life. So the drill instructor took his rifle stock and busted his toe and said, "That's your right foot; the one that hurts is the one you start with." Also, thirty years ago you could make a good living with your hands. A lot of these guys set up their own machine shop or they worked for the railroad. An inordinately high number of them are truck drivers because it's solitary. Mr. Jones is a truck driver. The guy couldn't read a lick. But he got around— just figured out his route and made sure the road signs and maps and addresses all matched. It's just phenomenal, the coping skills.

Q: Do you have evidence that your program makes a difference for inmates once they leave the prison?

SWANSON: The corrections department is in the midst of tracking outcomes—looking at, if we mandate education, will it result in less recidivism? As money gets tighter, they're going to want to go to the legislature and say, "Look, these people with these literacy skills have less recidivism." The cost for incarcerating somebody is between $30,000 and $50,000 per year. And the numbers are compounded for re-offenders because of the additional court costs. So the argument is, let's put maybe one-tenth of that money into a program prior to release to see if we can change that outcome.

Q: Why did you choose the Wilson Reading System?

SWANSON: I liked the fact that it integrates decoding and phonemic awareness, which a lot of reading programs don't. It's very explicit. There are three key neurological aspects to reading—decoding, isolating groups of letters into chunks, and automaticity. Wilson provides you with the reading, the writing, the placement, and the practice. Sometimes, a teacher will say, "He can read just fine." What that teacher may not know is that the student has this vast sight-word vocabulary imprinted on his brain, and he can recognize all these words. He's memorized a lot of words and he's great at context clues. But he can't decode unfamiliar words.

Q: What's your biggest reward teaching here?

SWANSON: When guys like Mr. O'Riley write a letter. He's severely disabled with a communication disorder and a mental-health problem. Learning to write was a huge struggle for him. And he said, "You know, I wrote my dad a letter before he died, and I'd never written my dad a letter before in my life. That was worth whatever I've had to do."

"TODAY, WE'RE GOING TO LEARN HOW TO MAKE COTTAGE CHEESE"

William was born in central Oregon with more than a few troubles. Besides being epileptic and bipolar, he got knocked around emotionally by unsup-

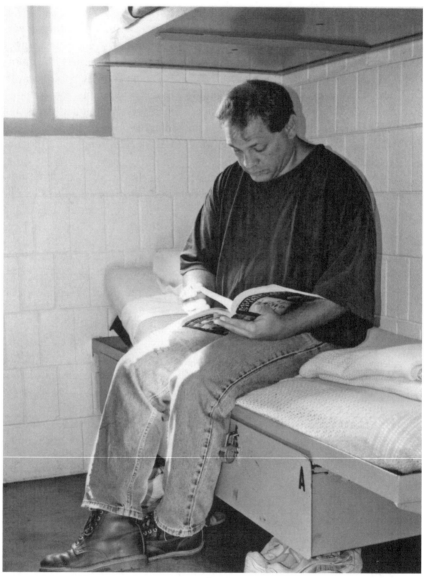

William

portive parents. It didn't help that the special-ed track where he spent his school years was missing at least one critical element: a reading and writing curriculum. It wasn't until William was a high school junior that a teacher picked up on a telltale clue to his learning problems: He kept reversing his *b*'s and *d*'s, *p*'s and *q*'s. That's when his dyslexia was, at last, diagnosed. But by then, William figured his illiteracy had solidified, like the lava that flowed, eons ago, in molten rivers across the central Oregon landscape.

What the public schools failed to do for him, however, the penitentiary did. When he landed at the Eastern Oregon Correctional Institution at age thirty-seven, he signed up for the horticulture program. He found himself learning all kinds of things about the classification and propagation of plants. "If I can learn about plants," he thought, "I can learn about anything."

This realization gave him the courage to jump into the special services program, where he methodically tackled the Wilson Reading System with help from inmate tutors. Less than a year later, this man who thought he would never crack a book can be found most evenings propped on his cot, lost in the pages of a Louis L'Amour western or a Stephen King horror story. At the time of this interview, his GED was nearly complete.

Q: Talk about your experience in the special-ed program at your public school.

WILLIAM: In special ed, basically, you did little assignments, like, "Today we're going to learn how to make cottage cheese." It was nothing to do with education, period. Not too many teachers were real thrilled about special ed.

Q: Were you in special ed all day long?

WILLIAM: I was in special ed for almost all seven periods of my classes.

Q: What else did you do beside make cottage cheese?

WILLIAM: We went on field trips and stuff. But, basically, the teachers were spending time with the people that needed more special treatment.

Q: The students with more severe disabilities?

WILLIAM: Yeah, the ones that were worse off. The teachers weren't really teaching the kids how to read or write. The main thing that they taught was, like, wood shop, small engines, mechanics, welding. That's what they knew I could do with my hands, so they put me in them areas that I was good at, where they had some type of trade. When I got into junior high and high school, I kept asking to learn how to read or say my ABCs, and nobody would teach me. When I finally turned eighteen, I learned how to say my ABCs.

Q: How did you learn?

WILLIAM: A friend of mine taught me.

Q: How did you feel about yourself all those years?

WILLIAM: Basically, I thought that everyone had proven my dad's theory right, that I was stupid and dumb, and I didn't know anything, right from wrong.

Q: Your dad put you down?

WILLIAM: My whole family did.

Q: How did it feel when you were told you were dyslexic?

WILLIAM: At first for me it was discouraging because everything was confirmed. My dad was right, my family was right, schoolteachers were right. OK, they win. Plus on top of that, my epilepsy, plus the mental illnesses that I have—it was like, everything was confirmed. OK, they win; I'm done.

Q: So you came to believe you were stupid?

WILLIAM: Well, now I don't. But I did at the time. I was very severely depressed, and pretty much I didn't have no self-confidence. Three months before my graduation, I walked out the door.

Q: When you came here and enrolled in the Wilson Reading System, you knew the alphabet, so you started from there?

WILLIAM: Yeah, I started working my way up. Now I can't put down a book, hardly. I sit there and I read anywhere from 200 to 600 pages a day.

Q: What do you like to read?

WILLIAM: Westerns, horror, romances. I read a little bit of everything.

Q: Does that change how you feel about yourself?

WILLIAM: It gives me more confidence. I can read something that gives me kind of a picture of what's going on. Before, if somebody told me, "OK, read this," then I would just guess.

Q: Once you left home, how did you cope with not being able to read? How did you do everyday reading, like signs and pill bottles?

WILLIAM: I asked somebody, "What does that say?" It gets embarrassing after a while.

Q: What do you want to do when you get out of here?

WILLIAM: I would like to take college. I like computers a lot—maybe do some computer programming.

"I FLUNKED FIRST GRADE, RIGHT OFF THE TOP"

Dale grew up dirt poor in a ramshackle house on Cooper Mountain, five miles from the school he attended in the Portland suburb of Tigard. The wages from his parents' low-skilled jobs didn't cover even the basics, like decent clothes

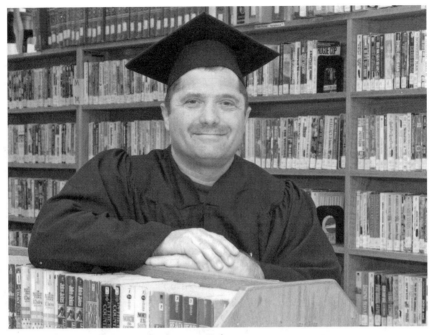

Dale

or hot water. As he struggled along, year after year—his raggedy mien drawing derision from his designer-label classmates—Dale's learning disability went undiagnosed. When he dropped out in ninth grade, he couldn't read a word.

After that, he survived by his wits, carefully guarding the secret of his illiteracy from his employers and from his three children. It gnawed at him, though, and he eventually sought out a tutor for reading instruction. But his good intentions crumbled when his marriage fell apart a few months later. Ironically, when the bars slammed shut behind him at Eastern Oregon Correctional Institution, thirty-nine-year-old Dale finally got the help and appropriate instruction in reading that had eluded him for a lifetime.

Q: What were your early years at school like?

DALE: I didn't fit in. Period. When I first started in school, in order to take a shower, we had to heat water on the stove, so we didn't get showers every day like other kids. I was considered a dirty kid. I was teased really bad. And my parents never showed me how to read and write. That just wasn't part of our lifestyle. I don't, to this day, even know if they knew how to read.

Q: So school was pretty miserable for you.

DALE: It was terrible. Here's a good start for you: I failed first grade. That's how good school was for me. I flunked first grade, right off the top. I finally made it to junior high and they had a class in the special-ed department. So here I am, I can't read and write. I'm embarrassed to even be in school, so what they did is got me a part-time job working at Tom's Pancake House. I went to school for a couple of hours in the morning and I worked all afternoon, and that was my school. Didn't know how to read and write, and they said: "Oh, you're doing great. You just passed the eighth grade, so now you're back up to ninth grade where you belong." And they shipped me off to high school. That didn't work. I left school in ninth grade.

Q: You never got the academic support you needed.

DALE: I started working, got married, had three kids, made it ten years without anybody really knowing I didn't know how to read. I worked at a gas station as a manager for almost three and a half years and couldn't read or write a bit, but I could do math all right. I can add and subtract, and I sure can count money. Nobody had a clue I couldn't read or write—no one. If it was something to do with reading, I'd just quit rather than say, "I've got a disability and I can't do this." I hid from it, you know. My kids would say, "Dad, read this." I'd say, "Not right now, later." And I just kept putting it off and putting it off to keep them from knowing that I couldn't read.

Q: How did you keep the secret?

DALE: Well, my wife knew. She helped me with that. After the divorce, my mother-in-law did my applications for jobs and such, because she knew. I'd pick up an application and say, "I ain't got time to do this right now, can I bring it back?" So I'd take the applications, she'd fill them out, then I would take them back. They had no clue.

Q: So you were faking it.

DALE: Yeah. You know, it amazes me now how well I got away with it. I was a hard worker; everybody loved the way I worked. I can do anything. I'm real intelligent as far as doing things, you know. I can rebuild cars, because I didn't need to read to do that. A couple of months before I got divorced, I decided, you know, they have all these places you can call that people will help you learn how to read, and I thought I'd really like to do that. I found a lady who volunteered her time at the library. She started teaching me, one-on-one. It lasted probably five or six months. I really looked forward to going up there and spending that time and getting the opportunity to read. And all of a sudden, here comes the divorce, so that was out. I couldn't concentrate. My wife took my kids, and I was very unhappy about that. I ended up in trouble and came here.

Q: It seems like you were able to turn your prison term into an opportunity.

DALE: This brought on a whole new life for me. One of the first things they ask you when you come to prison is, "What would you like to accomplish here?" I said, "I'd like to get my teeth fixed and I'd like to go to school." When I first got to the classroom, I was shy and I stood in the back of the class because I had no idea that this place could help me at all. They started working with me and I was having a real hard time with it, but one step led to another, and you know, I started thinking, "This just might work." I got through Level A, B, C, and D in reading. I've taken all four of the GED tests in the last year. And, you know, what an accomplishment, because I never thought it would ever come—ever. I did one and I said, "What do you mean I passed it?" So in the last five years, I've came a long ways.

Q: So you started out being a nonreader and you're almost done with your GED now?

DALE: Right. I've already passed science. I passed the essay and the reading. I've passed social studies, and the only one I have left is math. And I read books all the time now. My whole life is different. It was really good to write to my family. I had to apologize to them for the person that I was. I didn't know who I was because I didn't know myself. I'll be doing some college courses when I'm done with this.

Q: What do you like to read?

DALE: Everything. I've read *Little House on the Prairie*. I've read *Where the Red Fern Grows*. Just tons of them—*The Summer of the Monkeys*, all the Harry Potters. I just got done reading the fifth Harry Potter. I was second on the list waiting for that. It's just been a real pleasure for me. I can't thank this place enough. As far as I'm concerned, I'm happy I came here. I had to keep trying to find out the missing piece, and the missing piece was my illiteracy.

4

Bringing Reason to Reading:
What Modern Science Reveals

Studies once they hit paper look so clean, uncontroversial, and devoid of feelings.

—Linnea Ehri
Scientific Studies of Reading, 1998

Sadly, scientific research about what works does not usually find its way into most classrooms.

—Paula J. Stanovich and Keith E. Stanovich
Using Research and Reason in Education, 2003

There is in the field of education a difference between ideologically based sentiments about human nature and scientifically based knowledge about the human mind.

—E. D. Hirsch
Principal Leadership, 2003

Virginia Berninger fiddles with a laptop in the Clinical Training Lab as her ten graduate students in school psychology drift in for the first session of their course in educational neuropsychology. The University of Washington professor, who is as comfortable with the supersophisticated brain-imaging technologies she uses in her research as most people are with their microwave oven, is, ironically, stymied by the balky computer on the table in front of her. "How do you wake this thing up?" she wonders aloud. A couple of tech-savvy students jump up to help.

116

The computer malfunction ends up as a teachable moment—one that perfectly meshes with the course's content on reading disability. The department's techies, it turns out, had neglected to give Berninger the code for keeping the laptop running. "That's just what happens to dyslexic kids in the classroom," she tells her students. "They *can* learn to read, but they don't get the alphabetic code by osmosis. They need someone to reveal it to them directly. Communication of the code—that's the solution to the reading glitch."

When she finally gets her PowerPoint rolling and launches into what for her is household terminology—genotypes and neurotransmitters, the inferior frontal gyrus and the right cerebellum, the "phonological loop" and the "word-form area"—Berninger is in her element, drawing upon her decades of pioneering research on the cerebral and genetic links to the diagnosis and treatment of learning disabilities. Ensconced within the fortress-like brick walls of Miller Hall, the professor and her protégées are oblivious to the violent thunderstorm crashing and rumbling outside, unaware that on this very afternoon in late March, lightning is striking the city's legendary Space Needle just across Union Bay—a rare enough event to make the local five o'clock news.

Berninger's shoulder-length silver hair and deep-red velvet pantsuit sets her apart visually from her twenty- and thirty-something students, who are clad in the near-universal uniform of this rain-soaked city: blue jeans, natural fibers in earthy hues, fleece, Gore-Tex, waterproof boots. But the easy rapport between Berninger and her students quickly blurs differences of age and fashion and professional stature. In an atmosphere that is relaxed yet intellectually engaging, Berninger leads a lively dialogue, constantly lobbing questions to her students as she talks.

She dives into her topic with the passion that drives her work. "It's a criminal shame," she tells the aspiring school psychologists, "that teachers, who are in charge of learning in the classroom, get no formal training in the brain. They get *nothing*."

After class, she confides to us that she has volunteered to teach the same course content to preservice teachers at UW, but her offer has been turned down. "Neuropsychology doesn't mesh with the latest philosophical movement in education, which is constructivism," Berninger explains. "According to the constructivist philosophy, teachers don't tell students anything. The students are at the mercy of discovering it on their own as they construct their own meaning." She sees the current enthusiasm for constructivism as just another iteration—what she calls a "reincarnation"—of whole language, another spin of the ever-turning wheel of reading-philosophy birth and rebirth. (With whole language undergoing scrutiny in the public spotlight lately, the movement may well be trying to deflect attention with a little semantic sleight-of-hand.)

Berninger's 500-level seminar, like the field of reading itself, walks a delicate balance between hard science and humanism. With one breath, she talks about the spongy gray matter that rests inside the human cranium, and with the next she tells of anguished phone calls from parents whose children are floundering in school. (One family, for instance, sought her help after their dyslexic son's suicide attempt made his desperation undeniable.) One minute, she's pointing out the linkage of single-word reading skills to a region on chromosome 15. The next, she's talking about the sociopolitical issues that have impeded progress in the teaching of reading.

Just as the skills-versus-meaning dichotomy plagues the reading debate, the discipline of educational psychology is divided on a related quarrel: brain versus mind, and whether scientific research has relevance in teacher training and educational practice. Some scholars argue that the mind is transcendent, that the processes of thinking and learning are in truth much loftier than the lowly firings of neurons and the effects of neurotransmitters on neural pathways. But these sorts of metaphysical questions about the nature of the human mind rightly belong within the realms of philosophy and religion. In the realm of science, researchers like Berninger explain the brain-mind connection as simply two aspects of an integrated, physical system. "The mind," she says, "is the brain's activity, generated as it interacts with the internal and external environment."

Inexplicably, the same liberal educators who wouldn't dream of questioning the validity of brain-imaging technologies to detect Alzheimer's disease are deeply skeptical when scientists, using the very same high-powered machines to study the brain activity of struggling readers, find clear anomalies in these kids' language-processing brain mechanisms. The widespread denial in education circles that learning disabilities such as dyslexia can be traced to the anatomy and functioning of the brain is incomprehensible to Berninger, knowing as she does that 15,000 genes—fully half of the 30,000 genes that make us human—are expressed in the brain. After all, we are now well beyond the 1990s, which the federal government dubbed the "decade of the brain," with its explosion of discoveries about the complexities of the learning process. But the form-function duality in education seems to be coated in Teflon: The ever-mounting evidence about the neurological origins of dyslexia just doesn't stick when it comes to classroom practice.

WHERE FACTS AND FAITH COLLIDE

Berninger is exasperated by the political and philosophical infighting that has crippled discourse. In certain quarters, she reveals, the very ethics of studying how learning occurs in the brain have been questioned. Berninger describes an educational conference she attended where brain researchers were branded as unethical by a major education theorist. "You *have* to separate science from politics, and politics from education," she tells us. "You can't make any assumptions about a researcher's politics or ethics based on the nature of his or her research. Nor can you make assumptions about teachers' effectiveness based on their teaching philosophies."

Professor Berninger is baffled by another enduring myth: that researchers are trying to advance the pinched view that phonics is the be-all and end-all of reading instruction. That simply is not the case, she says. Citing the findings of the National Reading Panel, Berninger acknowledges that scientific research does indeed support the need to teach phonics, also known as the alphabetic principle or code (how letters stand for sounds). But science also points unequivocally to the necessity of teaching four other aspects of literacy, directly and explicitly: awareness of the sounds (phonemes) of spoken words, fluency (smooth, coordinated, and fast reading), vocabulary, and comprehension (meaning). Berninger's research program over the past twenty years is grounded in combining elements of whole language with an array of other elements based on scientific findings on listening, speaking, reading, and writing.

Critics who, with a reflexive jerk of the knee, reject the science of reading may well fail to notice that researchers such as Berninger have *never* doubted the educational value of literature, engaging stories, and high-interest content. Nor has research slighted the importance of meaning, or brushed off the indispensability of good teaching in any program of reading instruction. The polarized worldview that pits science against what Berninger calls a "politically correct philosophy" inhibits the kind of interdisciplinary study that is essential in a field as complex as reading.

"While some educators grasp this synthesis of the professional craft of educators with scientific research from the fields of psychology, linguistics, and neuroscience," Berninger observes, "others do not." Among the big losers is the profession itself. "What we are trying to do," she says, "is not only use science to identify effective instruction for all kinds of learners but also to raise the status of the teaching profession in the eyes of our society."

There's yet another chronic bias that puts teaching at loggerheads with research: the antipsychology stance that is widely taken in American education. Many education professionals reject not just the methods of science but the entire field of psychology. In fact, this posture seems equal in its fury to that of the most ferocious phonics foes. In a tone betraying both frustration and mystification, Berninger reports that the education profession seems to have a "vendetta" against psychologists. "It's really a kind of hatred," she reveals.

The present authors ran into this attitude a few years ago after we wrote a series of articles about the benefits of phonics for LD kids. The day the series hit the mailboxes of our readers, a flaming e-mail popped up in our inbox. It was from one of our former colleagues, and she was livid. Taking angry swipes at the Religious Right and its antihumanistic agenda, this normally even-tempered and reasonable woman complained bitterly, "The Religious Right thinks phonics is a cure for everything from sniffles to divorce." On top of that, she snarled, our series had quoted the writings of top reading researchers who hold doctorates, not in education, but in *psychology*. If an e-mail could sputter, this one would have. Its tone suggested that a PhD in psychology no more qualifies a person to conduct research in learning than a background in, say, astrology.

Since receiving that poison-pen message in 2003, we've encountered this attitude over and over. The psychology connection of today's reading-research community is one of the things that most irks whole-language advocates and the teacher trainers who have adopted the constructivist view. Many whole-language apologists, for example, disparage the reading research funded by the National Institutes of Health (NIH) in large part because it was led by G. Reid Lyon, whose expertise includes neurobiology and psychology as well as education, and because it is carried out by university-based researchers such as Berninger, who specialize in fields such as neuropsychology. They snubbed the National Reading Panel and the Committee on the Prevention of Reading Difficulties, too, whose seminal reports were written by eminent experts from many education-related fields, including the cognitive sciences and experimental psychology.

Given so many educators' enmity toward psychologists, it is ironic to note that two of the most pivotal progressive theorists whose ideas fed into the whole-language movement and child-centered education—John Dewey and Jean Piaget—were professors who taught and studied psychology. Both men were wholehearted proponents of testing educational theories by experimental means. Indeed, Dewey, whose first book was titled simply *Psychology*, was a protégé of prominent experimental psychologist G. Stanley Hall, who exerted a potent influence on Dewey's thinking. Jean Piaget, the exalted father of active learning, was also a staunch advocate of experimental methods.

It's perplexing, then, that the same progressive educators who are deeply beholden to the ideas of Dewey and Piaget complain that current research on reading is too heavily weighted toward the experimental methods of science in general, and of psychology in particular. We suggest that Dewey and Piaget would be displeased by the uncritical acceptance of whole language by American educators, as well as with the rejection of scientific evidence supporting phonics. By overlooking or minimizing the pro-experimental positions of these popular educational theorists, educators are guilty of selective reading of the scholars' works.

Here's what Piaget wrote in a statement titled *Education and Teaching since 1935*, published in the 1960s:

> Whether educational programs and teaching methods are imposed by the state or left to the initiative of teachers, it is still quite clear that we can make no justified statements about their practical productivity, or, above all, about the numerous unexpected effects that they may have upon the general formation of individuals, without systematic study employing all the means so fertile with possibilities for cross-checking that have been developed by modern statistical science and the various fields of psychosociological research. (1969, 20)

Piaget then went on to give an apt blueprint for settling the reading wars:

> It is, for example, a question for experimental pedagogy to decide whether the best way of learning to read consists in beginning with the letters, then graduating to words and finally to sentences, in accordance with the classical or "analytical" method, or whether it is better to work through these stages in reverse order, in accordance with Decroly's "total" method. Only a patient, methodical research program, using comparable groups of subjects for equally comparable periods of time, while taking care to neutralize as far as possible any adventitious factors (quality of the teachers and their preferences for one or other method, etc.), can permit a solution of the question. (1969, 21)

Piaget also hailed the power and importance of interdisciplinary study. Here's what he said about that: "Any advances to be made by experimental pedagogy, taken as an independent science with regard to its subject matter, must necessarily be linked, as in all sciences, to interdisciplinary researches, if there is to be any question of constituting it as a true science—of its being, in other words, not merely descriptive but explanatory" (1969, 24).

Professor Dewey (who, incidentally, after earning his PhD in philosophy, retreated behind the ivy halls of academe after teaching in a public high school for only two years) also lauded experimental psychology. Somewhat alarmed by the progressive educational movement spawned by his theories, Dewey sought to rein in some of the excesses in his 1938 statement, *Experience and Education*. He takes a somewhat scolding tone when he says this:

> Those who are looking ahead to a new movement in education, adapted to the existing need for a new social order, should think in terms of Education itself rather than in terms of some 'ism about education, even such an 'ism as "progressivism." For in spite of itself any movement that thinks and acts in terms of an 'ism becomes so involved in reaction against other 'isms that it is unwittingly controlled by them. For

it then forms its principles by reaction against them instead of by a comprehensive, constructive survey of actual needs, problems, and possibilities. (6)

And this: "It is not too much to say that an educational philosophy which professes to be based on the idea of freedom may become as dogmatic as ever was the traditional education which is reacted against. For any theory and set of practices is dogmatic which is not based upon critical examination of its own underlying principles" (1938, 22).

In introducing Dewey's book, Alfred L. Hall-Quest, editor of Kappa Delta Pi Publications, wrote the following:

> *Education and Experience* is a lucid analysis of both "traditional" and "progressive" education. The fundamental defects of each are here described. Where the traditional school relied upon subjects or the cultural heritage for its content, the "new" school has exalted the learner's impulse and interest and the current problems of a changing society. Neither of these sets of values is sufficient unto itself. *Both* are essential. (Dewey 1938, 9–10)

How so many educators can embrace the progressive legacies of Dewey and Piaget with respect to classroom practice while rejecting experimental methods applied to educational problems is one of the riddles of the reading wars. Dewey's cautionary words against clinging mindlessly to 'isms and dogmas have been ignored.

Faith-Based Teaching

Educators who deny the science of reading have put themselves in an untenable position. It's a position that is, at its heart, a fundamentalist position. It's the attitudinal petrifaction that allows people to deny hard evidence whenever that evidence contradicts their belief system. The whole-language fundamentalists, girded in the armor of righteousness, attack the rigorous scientific research on reading coming from more than fifty major research institutions in the United States, as well as others throughout the world. They reject findings from psychology, neurology, and medicine which, they argue, should stay inside their own disciplines and quit meddling in the field of education.

In the debate about reading, the so-called progressive and conservative positions have been flipped on their heads. Phonics, embraced by religious conservatives who are often loath to buy into a rationalistic understanding of things, is in fact the scientifically supportable position. Some might argue that, in this instance, conservatives are exploiting science in a cynical scheme to promote their true agenda, a "back-to-basics" movement that rejects critical thinking, creativity, innovation, discovery learning, and child-centered methods. But that argument, Berninger asserts, is "overly simplistic and potentially misleading." In reality, it's the inability—or unwillingness—of progressive educators to separate the legitimate science from the big, squirming can of political and religious worms that has stalled progress in the field of reading.

In the topsy-turvy reading wars, progressives have too often been the ideologues, clinging stubbornly to an increasingly repudiated position solely on faith. For countless educators, this faith in holistic instruction—whether you call it whole language or try to give it new respectability with an Orwellian rechristening—continues to eclipse the emerging body of evidence that has, study by study, decade by decade, made Swiss cheese of the assumptions of Kenneth Goodman and his followers.

"I don't know why education, and in particular reading, within the field of education, has been so wimpy with respect to building on evidence rather than on heart," Reid Lyon muses in his 2004 interview with Children of the Code. If Professor Berninger successfully meets her learning objectives for her course in educational neuropsychology, her students will use both—their heads *and* their hearts—when, as school psychologists, they work toward excellent learning outcomes for all of their students. She envisions a field full of "scientist practitioners," educators who can draw competently and compassionately upon *all* the evidence—evidence about the brain, about reading development, about the emotional underpinnings of learning—in designing and assessing reading interventions that really work. This new generation of educators will then be able to bolster students' emotional well-being along with their reading achievement.

THE CASE FOR SCIENCE

The education researchers who are doing clinical trials and field studies on reading are equivalent to medical researchers whose discoveries in the laboratory end up saving lives in doctor's offices and hospitals. Basic science informs practice in medicine. When educators wall themselves off from experts in related fields, wedded to a don't-confuse-me-with-the-facts ideology, questions about professional malfeasance arise. Can a teacher reject or ignore findings that impinge directly on her practice, yet still claim, credibly, to be an informed, competent, effective professional? To use a medical analogy, you probably wouldn't want to be treated by a doctor who didn't read medical journals. To this, you might respond, "Yeah, but medicine is different from education." True. But the scientific method is the same, no matter what the field of investigation.

Teachers should, like physicians, welcome any evidence that impinges upon their practice as a boon, not a butt-in. To reject what Lyon calls the "multidisciplinary research teams [that] study cognitive, linguistic, neurobiological, genetic, and instructional factors related to early reading development and reading difficulties" (1998, 15) is to reject the belief that learning is an infinitely complex process that is both physical and psychological, both biological and sociological, both brain based and classroom based.

The NIH research began focusing in the mid-1980s on closing knowledge gaps in four areas: What does it take to learn to read? What goes wrong when you don't? How do you prevent it? And how do you remediate it? "There's no way to answer those four questions," Lyon says, "unless you have neurologists on board, pediatricians on board, neuroscientists on board, educators on board, cognitive neuroscientists on board" (2004).

The Scientific Method: So What?

There was a popular psychology professor at Portland State University in the 1970s who packed in the freshmen for his Psych 101 class. With his wild hair and holey jeans, Professor Maynard would sit on a table before the roomful of impressionable eighteen-year-olds who were in awe of his braininess and, even more, his bohemian aura. The surprising thing about the professor's Intro to Psychology course was the way he launched the topic: His first several lessons focused on the scientific method—what it is, and why it matters so much, not only in the "hard" sciences of chemistry and biology and physics and medicine but also in the human sciences. The rigorous methods of science, Maynard insisted, are what give validity and reliability to all claims of knowledge.

Why did this psych guy put so much effort into enlightening a bunch of freshmen on the scientific method, when they had signed up for lectures on human behavior? Our guess is that the professor knew that his liberal arts students might not get another chance to hear the pitch for scientific rigor as they pursued their degrees in fields such as English literature or art history or elementary education. Others, he was aware, would drop out or drift away to take jobs and raise families and would, as voters and community members, profit from some understanding of the methods of science that underpin human progress in such practical and pressing matters as the prevention and treatment of disease, including the development of safe and effective pharmaceuticals. Or the gathering danger of pollution and the development of strategies for environmental protection. Or the mysteries of deep space and the secrets of the human psyche.

Without an understanding of scientific method, Maynard's students, as they ventured out into the world, would have no sure means of discerning objective truth from speculation, superstition, supposition, opinion, religion, or outright deception. We suspect that Professor Maynard grabbed his chance to convey the message that, in an age of reason, science is the means by which we answer the question, How do you know?

Scientific method hinges on verification. The accumulation of clues that, over time, support a certain conclusion is called a "preponderance of evidence." The scientist is a skeptic. She wants to know exactly how you gathered your data and arrived at your conclusion so she can replicate your study in order to prove—or disprove—your claims for herself. You publish your findings, she publishes her findings, other researchers review the work, and little by little, a critical mass of evidence builds up. After testing, refining, narrowing down, retesting, researchers in a given field can say, "We know, with a great deal of certainty, that A causes B, or method Y works better than method X." (Science never rests its case completely, because the very nature of science is to prop open the door to new findings.)

The evidence on teaching reading is there, and has been building for decades. Yet it has not been embraced by the educational mainstream. "Educational practice has suffered greatly because its dominant model for resolving or adjudicating disputes has been more political (with its corresponding factions and interest groups) than scientific," Stanovich and Stanovich say (2003, 5).

At its core, the reading debate is really a clash about "ways of knowing." Daniel Hallahan of the University of Virginia and Cecil Mercer of the University of Florida discuss this collision of ideas over the "nature of knowledge" within the historical context of the learning disabilities field, identifying (yet again) a competing pair of worldviews: modernism and postmodernism.

"The modern position supports the use of scientific method of inquiry to increase knowledge and features experimental research designs and quantitative methods," Hallahan and Mercer write. "Postmodernism rejects the modern view of science in favor of alternative ways of knowing. Postmodernism primarily supports a socially constructed view of knowledge in which logical inquiry is a social enterprise" (2002, 399).

The authors go on to assert, "Critics of postmodernism . . . maintain that the most questionable tenet of postmodernism is the rejection of science because it is thought of as untrustworthy or evil. The concern emerges because the rejection of science insulates socially constructed knowledge from compelling criticism and allows points of view to be endorsed that promote agendas that could be scientifically challenged" (Hallahan and Mercer 2002, 399).

As National Reading Panel member Joanne Yatvin noted in her letter criticizing the panel's report, teachers who are subject to legislative mandates are very unhappy about losing their *"authority to decide what is best for their students"* (National Reading Panel 2000, italics added). Science's answer to that complaint is this: Authority resides in verifiable knowledge. Knowing, for the scientist, is based on a public record, a body of literature, a shared accumulation of data, and ongoing critical analysis by peers. It's not based on artistry or talent or intuition or what *seems* right or what *feels* right in your heart or what you *wish* were right in the best of all possible worlds.

Nor does authority derive from a handout from murky origins, no matter how widely disseminated it might be, no matter how many times it has turned up in workshop packets or PowerPoints at school-district in-services. Just because a piece of information is out there, everywhere, doesn't mean it has intellectual weight. Just because the latest rift between Ben and J-Lo or between Jen and Brad makes the five o'clock news in every major market across the United States doesn't mean the story is legitimate journalism.

Marilyn Jager Adams did some academic detective work in the late 1990s, looking into the origins of one such ubiquitous handout: a Venn diagram depicting whole language's "three-cueing system." Despite having no known author, the graphic—a trio of overlapping circles showing the essential elements for creating meaning in reading—had gotten a firm foothold among the community of reading teachers (1998, 73–99). Yet Adams, whose knowledge of the reading process is as comprehensive as anyone's in America, had never run into it until she started traveling the country to talk with teachers about reading research.

Here's how Louisa Cook Moats explains the "three-cueing" concept:

> Whole language dictates that recognition of unknown words is a function of three "cueing systems." Semantic, syntactic, and graphophonic processes are depicted as the enablers of functional reading, although the graphophonic cueing system (an invention of whole language, not of cognitive psychology) plays a minor, back-up role in whole-language models of reading. The sense of the passage is supposed to drive word recognition. The graphophonic cueing system is to be deployed as a strategy of last resort if context-based guessing has not yielded the correct word. The problem with the model, however, is that skilled readers do not rely on context to read words. They recognize them out of context by their letter-sound correspondences. (2000, 5)

Even though practically every practitioner Adams ran into was familiar with the diagram, none of them knew where it had originated. After making inquiries as far away as New Zealand and Australia, Adams had to conclude that the three-cueing diagram had spread, unattributed, through the grassroots of the educational community. In the decades since its possible beginnings in a 1976 article in *Language Arts* by P. David Pearson (reprinted in 1983 by the International Reading Association), its interpretation and use have been hybridized—tainted with, in Adams's words, "simplifications and distortions." As it passed from workshop to workshop, curriculum framework to district training, the diagram's look and meaning morphed. It's like the old childhood game of Telegraph: The original message, after being whispered from ear to ear around a circle, is unrecognizable by the time it gets to the last player. As Adams discovered,

> The three-cueing schematic is sometimes presented as a rationale for subordinating the value of the graphophonemic information to syntax and semantics and, by extension, for minimizing and even eschewing attention to the teaching, learning, and use of the graphophonemic system. This interpretation directly contradicts the logical import of the Venn diagram which, by virtue of its structure, asserts that productive reading depends on the inter-working of all three systems. (1998, 79)

One major whole-language player, Regie Routman, has published the three-cueing diagram in her book *Invitations* (1994), adding her interpretation of the reading process to elevate semantic cues (context: what makes sense) and syntactic cues (structure and grammar: what sounds right), while greatly minimizing the importance of graphophonic cues (letter-sound relationships) in the teaching and learning of reading. For Routman, "phonics truly seems to be a last resort," Adams concludes in her 1998 paper, which she wrote as a visiting scholar at Harvard University Graduate School of Education. Adds Adams, "Routman's approach not only denies the utility of the alphabetic principle but fails to reveal its basic logic and structure" (84).

Unraveling the tortuous saga of the three-cueing diagram was, for Adams, a "sobering revelation" (1998, 90). This grassroots dissemination and near-universal adoption of an idea loosely rooted and grown wildly askew—without reference to a body of knowledge or a scholarly tradition or a chain of evidence—highlights, she says, "the profound breach in information and communication that separates the teaching and research communities" (90). Adams, who is now chief scientist at Soliloquy Learning and a visiting professor of cognitive and linguistic sciences at Brown University, laments:

> In the world of practice, the widespread subscription to the belief system that the three-cueing diagram has come to represent has wreaked disaster on students and hardship on teachers. At the same time, it is the underlying cause of not insignificant distrust and ill-will between teachers, teacher educators, and researchers. Yet, while teachers widely believe that the lore of the three-cueing system is based on the best of current research, researchers are barely aware of its existence, nature or influence. The lesson of this story is thus clear and urgent. We must work together to rebuild the bridge, socially and intellectually, between those involved in research and prac-

tice. Toward regaining respect for as well as the productivity, morale, and forward momentum of our educational system, there may be no more important effort we can undertake. (1998, 90)

This story and its plea for research and practice to join forces in no way denigrates or discounts the vital importance of craft knowledge in teaching or in any other profession, whether it be counseling troubled children or healing sick patients, piloting airplanes, or breeding dogs. The experience and independent judgment of practitioners will always matter hugely in decisions about a course of psychotherapy or chemotherapy, seat-of-the-pants flying in a hailstorm, or raising purebreds worthy of "best in show." Whichever reading method or curriculum is chosen, the teacher's skill will always be essential to its effectiveness.

The view among educators that teaching is not a science but an art—a creative endeavor that depends on the talent, intuition, resourcefulness, and, above all, the professional discretion of the teacher—is a formidable impediment to ending the reading wars. Instead of looking at evidence with the dispassionate eye of the scientist, teachers who are confronted with conflicting theories about reading often react as artists do—with their gut, coming down on the side that feels right. But once again, a false dichotomy has been set up, suggesting that craft and science are mutually exclusive. In fact, they buttress and bolster each other. "As with medicine," Stanovich and Stanovich stress, "constructing teaching practice on a firm scientific foundation does not mean denying the craft aspects of teaching" (2003, 3). Other writers share this view about teaching as art. David C. Berliner writes, "No one I know denies the artistic component to teaching. I now think, however, that such artistry should be research-based. I view medicine as an art, but I recognize that without its close ties to science it would be without success, status, or power in our society. Teaching, like medicine, is an art that also can be greatly enhanced by developing a close relationship to science" (Berliner 1987, 4).

P. David Pearson, too, cautioned against bucking science. In his 1999 review of the work of the Committee on the Prevention of Reading Difficulties for the National Research Council of the National Academy of Sciences, he warned that "hiding behind the 'art of teaching' defense will eventually threaten teacher autonomy. Teachers need creativity, but they also need to demonstrate that they know what evidence is, and that they recognize that they practice a profession based in behavioral science" (Stanovich and Stanovich, 33).

The observations of a gifted practitioner may well be the jumping-off point for science—the origins of a hypothesis that can then be tested and verified.

The initial studies in a field like education are often case studies or descriptive ethnographies—the "qualitative" research that characterizes the investigations typically done in whole language. These kinds of studies, researchers agree, have tremendous value. But they are not sufficient, in and of themselves, to answer the critical questions of cause and effect. To do that, a scientific investigation must also include "quantitative" research—experimental studies that isolate the various factors (in scientific parlance, the "variables") that can affect the result.

In their purest sense, experimental studies randomly create two (or three or four) groups, which are similar in basic characteristics (such as race, age, family background). Each group then receives a different "treatment"—in the present case, one group may receive whole-language instruction over a nine-month period, another may receive a phonics-heavy curriculum, and a third may get a combination of the two approaches. A fourth group may be designated as the "control" group, meaning they receive no special treatment at all. The ethics of social sciences, however, don't allow for the control group to receive a placebo—the equivalent of a sugar pill, zero intervention. You wouldn't, for example, send them out to the playground for a nine-month recess. So in educational experiments, the "control" group typically receives whatever instructional program is already in place at the school they attend— that is, they get what they would have gotten if the study weren't underway. In education research, logistics and economics are other barriers to conducting truly random studies in the field. That's why most studies to date have fallen into the category of "quasi experimental," or *almost* experimental. Although true randomization is rarely feasible, it is becoming more common as the public and policymakers demand more accountability from schools and curriculum companies.

The NIH's research on reading "integrates quantitative and qualitative methods to increase the richness, impact, and ecological validity of the data," Lyon wrote in *Education Leadership* in March 1998. "However, using qualitative research methods requires the same scientific rigor employed in quantitative studies" (15).

Stanovich and Stanovich offer this caution about qualitative studies:

The insights gained from case studies or qualitative investigations may be quite useful in the early stages of an investigation of a certain problem. They can help us determine which variables deserve more intense study. . . . However, when we move from the early stages of scientific investigation, where case studies may be very useful, to the more mature stages of theory testing—where adjudicating between causal explanations is the main task—the situation changes drastically. Case studies and qualitative description are not useful at the later stages of scientific investigation because they cannot be used to confirm or disconfirm a particular causal theory.

They lack the comparative information necessary to rule out alternative explanations. (2003, 22)

In other words, such research must be regarded as "preliminary/exploratory,
observational, hypothesis generating," according to Joel R. Levin of the University of Wisconsin and Angela M. O'Donnell of Rutgers University
(2000, 26).

Four decades ago, Charles Fries observed, wryly, that "the discussions of
methods and the published opinions of reading 'experts' seem often to ignore
the limitations given in the research studies themselves, and, in the spirit of
'science fiction,' project the claims to knowledge far beyond anything that
the studies are prepared to deliver" (1962, 4). With nothing less than the
future of a child at stake, why would teachers embrace claims that are not
backed by solid studies? Inexplicably, teachers "are often confronted with
the view (that) there are no ways to verify what works best, that teachers
should base their practice on intuition," Stanovich and Stanovich write.
"This provides a fertile environment for gurus to sell untested educational
'remedies' that are not supported by an established research base and, often,
to discredit science, scientific evidence, and the notion of research-based best
practice in education" (2003, 4–5).

THE PERRY MASON METHOD

You can think of the findings of reading researchers as the forensic evidence
in the reading controversy. In the U.S. criminal justice system, the prosecutor
presents a detailed accumulation of evidence to support a conviction. Some
of the evidence is circumstantial (time, place, motive) and other evidence is
physical (blood, DNA, fingerprints). Anybody who watches *Law and Order*
on TV or reads Ann Rule's true-crime stories knows that it's tough to get a
conviction on circumstantial evidence alone. That's because that sort of
"soft" evidence may *look* convincing on its face, but scratch the surface and
there may be countless competing explanations. It's too open to error or interpretation or bias. By the same token, most judges don't allow hearsay into
the courtroom. Just as the U.S. legal system protects citizens from a conviction based on "he said, she said" testimony, the school system needs to protect children from victimization by educational hearsay. When a so-called
reading expert comes along and says, "This is how kids learn to read," educators need to ask for the evidence. They need to ask, with skepticism, "How
do you know?"

DR. FRANKENSTEIN, I PRESUME?

Much of educators' distrust of using science-based methods in a humanistic field such as education can be summed up by a favorite wisecrack of a late colleague of ours at the nonprofit Northwest Regional Educational Laboratory. When acquaintances would ask Tony, "What in the heck is an 'educational laboratory'?" he would say, "It's where they have a bunch of tiny little kids in test tubes." The quirky image, which perfectly captured the apparent oxymoron, always got a laugh. Like a lot of humor, Tony's joke derived its punch from the discomfort—the psychic dissonance—it caused in his listeners.

Some of the chafing against education research comes, no doubt, from the enduring stereotype of science as a sterile enterprise involving test tubes and petri dishes, of scientists as cold and unswervingly clinical. Teachers are prone to regard researchers as remote and emotionless, dangerously removed from the realities of classrooms, locked in their ivory towers with no genuine feeling for, or understanding of, children.

"Some educators reject public, depersonalized knowledge in social science because they believe it dehumanizes people," Stanovich and Stanovich write (10). Many teachers think scientists should stick to studying bugs and greenhouse gases, and leave kids and classrooms alone. This fear of dehumanizing children, of reducing them to statistical ciphers, is, we believe, one of the biggest sources of resistance to using science to guide teaching.

Harvard Professor Jeanne Chall, who broke new ground in the field of reading, wrote that her "overriding impression" during her classic 1967 study was "one of strong emotional involvement" among authors, reading specialists, teachers, administrators, and even researchers. "Their language," she said, "was often more characteristic of religion and politics than of science and learning." She went on to note: "Visits to classrooms in particular impressed me with the ideological nature of the controversy. In general, I found emotion where reason should prevail" (7).

With sincere puzzlement, Chall asked in the updated version of her study, published in 1983, "How is it possible that during a time of growing research evidence, some of the statements on various issues of the debate seem as heated as in 1967—and in 1841?" She pleaded, once again, for "a more balanced rhetoric and use of research findings" (1983, introduction, 44).

She wrote those words more than twenty years ago. Yet the ideological skirmishes and theoretical firefights over reading instruction rage on. Lyon seems genuinely stumped about the reasons for the continuing salvos:

> The resistance in the educational community, particularly at the higher education level where teachers are trained, is enormous, almost unbelievable. When you show

people objective information, non-philosophically driven research—that for these kids, these interactions work very productively such that a youngster who was at the 10th percentile in reading before is now at the 60th percentile in reading—and you can show that time after time, but you still see substantial resistance from the educational community, it begins to tell us that many of these issues are way beyond the kids' issues, these are adult issues. They are fascinating adult issues where human beings are latching onto their beliefs, their assumptions, their egos, and their careers rather than looking very clearly at what works, what doesn't, making sure people know what works, measuring it, and getting the kids up to snuff. . . . We're in fact trying to study the factors that maintain these kinds of dichotomous thinking, where people polarize phonics/whole language, qualitative versus quantitative research. (2004)

THE TRUE BELIEVERS

The arguments of the whole-language camp are steeped in a "true believer" aura that runs counter to the tenets of liberalism: broadmindedness marked by questioning, intellectual curiosity, and forward thinking. The typical progressive educator, embracing the findings of the biological sciences, is likely to take the position that the demands of fundamentalist Christians who repudiate evolution and who want equal time for creationism in public school science classes are misplaced, at best. She probably believes, too, in the worldwide scientific consensus that carbon emissions from fossil fuels are warming the atmosphere and could lead, ultimately, to a global environmental disaster. But when it comes to the international scientific consensus on reading development and disability, this same progressive educator reacts with disbelief, even hostility. We are reminded of a fundamentalist neighbor who rejects the findings of paleontology and geology because the evidence of rocks and bones, pointing to eons of flux and evolution, contradicts scripture, which puts the genesis of planet Earth at about 6,000 years ago. We respect the sincerely held beliefs that allow devout people to take this kind of mystical leap over physical, tangible, provable evidence. But in the realm of education, faith and facts must be disentangled. And in reading, as in evolution, the question is the same: How do you know?

Philosopher Jonathan Adler, writing in the *Skeptical Inquirer* in January 1998, made this observation: "What truly marks an open-minded person is the willingness to follow where the evidence leads. The open-minded person is willing to defer to impartial investigations rather than to his own predilections. . . . Scientific method is attunement to the world, not to ourselves" (41).

TEN IMPORTANT FINDINGS ON READING

The National Institutes of Health's studies of normal reading development span forty years and six administrations, Democrat and Republican. NIH-supported researchers have studied more than 10,000 children, published more than 2,500 articles, and written more than fifty books that present the results of ten large-scale longitudinal studies and more than 1,500 smaller-scale experimental and cross-sectional studies. The U.S. Department of Education's Office of Educational Research and Improvement (now the Institute of Education Sciences) and Office of Special Education Programs, as well as the Canadian Research Council, have also contributed to the research base.

"The good news," Yale's Sally Shaywitz says, "is that data coming in from laboratories all over the world are providing a clear picture of the process of learning to read. Finally, a growing number of scientists, clinicians, and educators agree about what every child needs to know to become a good reader" (2003, 174).

Diving into this vast body of science, however, can be a chilling prospect. The off-putting opacity of scientific terminology is undoubtedly another reason that research has been sidelined in literacy circles. Admittedly, the average scientific report is as digestible as a bowl of cold sauerkraut. Fortunately, several recent publications have collected, analyzed, and summarized hundreds of articles, books, and reports in prose that is, if not exactly sparkling, at least not migraine-inducing. Taken together, the publications listed in the following section (p. 145) offer a broad overview of reliable research.

As a sampling, we've pulled together a few key findings that, based on converging evidence, have broad implications for reading instruction practices and policies. Our "Ten Important Findings" list gives just a brief taste of the scientific record on reading from the past three decades. It is meant only to whet the appetite for further reading. We have quoted heavily from the work of some of the most eloquent and impassioned voices in the current reading debate, among them Marilyn Adams of Soliloquy Learning and author of *Beginning to Read*; Virginia Berninger of the University of Washington; Linnea Ehri of the Graduate Center of the City University of New York; G. Reid Lyon, formerly of the National Institutes of Health, now with Dallas-based Best Associates; Sally Shaywitz of Yale University; Joseph Torgesen of Florida State University; Sharon Vaughn of the University of Texas at Austin; and the late Jeanne Chall, namesake of Harvard University's Graduate School of Education's literacy laboratory.

1. The Reading Disability Epidemic

The widely cited 1983 Connecticut study, done by Sally Shaywitz and Bennett Shaywitz, found that reading disability affects one child in five. "From a national perspective this means that there is not a family in America who has not been touched by a reading disability in some way," Sally Shaywitz writes. She goes on to bemoan the gaping chasm between the numbers of LD kids being served in schools versus the numbers of kids *needing* services. "In the Connecticut study," she says, "each child was administered a test of intelligence and a reading test individually. Using this methodology, we found that 20 percent of children were reading below their age, grade, or level of ability. . . . [Yet] less than one-third of the children who were reading below their age, ability, or grade level were receiving school services for their reading difficulty. This strongly suggested undiagnosed problems" (2003, 30).

But if you factor in all the kids who may not fall on the extreme end of the LD continuum—that is, those kids who don't have a biologically based reading glitch but have significant trouble learning to read—even the 20 percent figure may be too low. Reading tests nationwide "indicate that reading disability may be much more prevalent," says Shaywitz. She cites the "shocking data" coming from the National Assessment for Educational Progress (NAEP)—the "nation's report card"—such as the 2001 scores showing that nearly 40 percent of America's fourth-graders are unable to read at a fourth-grade level (2003, 29–30).

2. Reading by Guesswork

Research has revealed key facts related to Goodman's famous characterization of reading as a "psycholinguistic guessing game."

First, content words (as opposed to connecting words) can be predicted accurately from surrounding context only 10 percent to 20 percent of the time, researchers Philip B. Gough, Jack A. Alford, and Pamela Holley-Wilcox found in the early 1980s. Content words—nouns and verbs—are the words that do the heavy lifting in reading. It really doesn't do a reader much good to become an able guesser of pronouns, articles, or prepositions.

Second, it turns out that good readers don't guess anyway. It's only the struggling readers—that is, readers who don't know how to analyze words by pulling them apart and sounding them out—who resort to guessing. Adams has revealed in a series of studies that good readers focus on individual letters and groups of letters when they look at a page. She explains that because most good readers aren't aware of looking at distinct letters, it seems as if they're gleaning meaning in some sort of magical manner. She summarized these facts about word-recognition processes in skilled readers this way:

> It has been proven beyond any shade of doubt that skillful readers process virtually each and every word and letter of text as they read. This is extremely counterintuitive. For sure, skillful readers neither look nor feel as if that's what they do. But that's because they do it so quickly and effortlessly. Almost automatically, with almost no conscious attention whatsoever, skillful readers recognize words by drawing on deep and ready knowledge of spellings and their connections to speech and meaning. (1990b, 207)

Torgesen offers this explanation of how the reading process works:

> Skilled readers do not "skim and scan" text as they read for meaning, but rather they directly fixate and process a very high proportion of all the words in text. Furthermore, they accurately identify most of the words in text by processing information about all, or almost all, the letters in words. In other words, skilled word recognition is heavily dependent upon very detailed knowledge of the letters used to spell individual words. Skilled readers do not guess at the identity of specific words in text by relying on context; rather, they are able to accurately and fluently identify words on the basis of their written spellings. (2002, 10)

3. The Reading Brain

"The field of neuroscience is exploding," writes Sally Shaywitz who, as a physician specializing in learning disorders at Yale University, is among a handful of experts doing real-time imaging of brains wrestling with written words. "Recent advances in our understanding of the brain mechanisms underlying reading are nothing short of revolutionary" (2003, 6).

Lyon notes that researchers now understand that there are "specific systems in the brain" that "recover sounds from spoken words" (1998, 16). Shaywitz explains that the area at the back of the brain called the occipito-temporal zone is where skilled readers react "almost instantly to the whole word as a pattern." The reaction is so fast—less than 150 milliseconds—that it takes less time than a heartbeat, Shaywitz says. This region of the brain is known among reading researchers as the "word-form" area. "Careful examination of brain activation patterns has revealed a glitch in this circuitry in dyslexic readers," she says. "Studies from around the world leave no doubt that dyslexic readers use different brain pathways than do good readers" (2003, 78–79).

What's more, early intervention can alter these pathways. Citing a raft of research findings, Berninger says, "At least nine studies, using a range of imaging methodologies, including functional magnetic resonance imaging (fMRI), functional magnetic spectroscopic imaging (fMRS), magnetic source imaging (MSI) and electrophysiological recordings of event-related potentials (ERPs) now show that the brains of beginning readers, developing readers, and adults change in processing related to reading in normal and disabled readers" (2006). This phenomenon is what Shaywitz calls "brain repair." She writes, "It has now been shown that the brain can be rewired and that struggling children can become skilled readers" (2003, 86).

These findings, which should have hit the world of education like the thunderous splash of a calving glacier have, instead, impacted the field more like the plink of a lone raindrop. "Alas," says Shaywitz, "much of the time this new information appears to be a well-kept secret. In an era when we can image the brain as an individual reads and literally see the brain at work, it is unacceptable to have children and adults struggling to read when they could benefit from what modern neuroscience has taught us about reading and dyslexia" (2003, 6).

Shaywitz and Berninger are among the leaders in the race to untangle the neurological, genetic, and behavioral threads in reading disability. During her graduate seminar on educational neuropsychology, Berninger projects a slide labeled "The Brain on Book." She tells her students: "The anterior cyngulate goes *wild*. The dyslexic brain is in shock." Her University of Washington team, like the Yale team, uses imaging technologies to see what's happening inside the brain in vivo—that is, when it's alive—a profound improvement over the old days of dissecting the brains of cadavers.

The UW announced in May 2000 that this real-time imaging had revealed chemical differences in brain function of dyslexic and nondyslexic children during sound-processing tasks. Studies like this exemplify the new generation of education research, which rivals the rigor of medicine and other "hard" sciences.

In one UW study, fifteen ten- to thirteen-year-old boys in two matched groups—eight dyslexics and seven nondyslexics—participated in a yearlong treatment program designed by Berninger and her colleague Todd Richards to improve their skills in understanding and using the sounds of language. Reading instruction was blended into a hands-on workshop exploiting the boys' love of science. Images of their brains taken before and after the treatment found that the dyslexics' brain chemistry had changed significantly. At first, they used about four times the brain energy of their nondisabled counterparts to process sounds. Afterward, they used only 1.8 times the brain energy—a huge leap in efficiency. The dyslexics also made big gains in reading. They all started out well below grade level. Yet by the end, all but one could read grade-appropriate passages. "This research offers a message of hope," Berninger said in 2000 when the findings were released. "Parents of the boys in the study told us that children who didn't read independently before are now picking up books on their own and reading them" (University of Washington Office of News and Information).

The discovery that dyslexia is neurobiological in origin has given great comfort to dyslexic children and their families. Brain research has shot down the conventional wisdom that if you can't read, you must be lazy or obstinate or, worst of all, stupid. But there is still much more work to be done to unravel the Gordian knot of genetics and neurology that impinge upon the complex behavior we call reading.

4. The "Big Ideas" of Reading

Research has pinpointed five key skills needed for learning to read in English: (1) phonemic awareness, (2) alphabetic principle (phonics), (3) fluency, (4) vocabulary, and (5) comprehension. University of Oregon researchers call these the "big ideas" in beginning reading. (The National Reading Panel also identified the same five elements, but organized the skills a little differently in its report. The panel grouped phonemic awareness and phonics underneath the umbrella of the alphabetic principle, and grouped vocabulary instruction with comprehension strategies.)

The first big idea—*phonemic awareness* (being able to distinguish and identify the separate sounds in spoken words)—requires nothing less than "linguistic gymnastics," Lyon asserts, because the brain has to "pull from that one burble or acoustic bundle the three (or more) separate sounds. The ear never hears the individual sounds unless we spell them out." Lyon goes on to say, "Phonemic awareness is absolutely critical, non-negotiable to understanding how to read, to knowing how to bring sound to print because we have an alphabetic language, [but] it is in no way sufficient" (2004).

The second big idea—*the alphabetic principle*—draws the loudest salvos in the reading wars because understanding the alphabetic principle is what phonics is all about. Learning to read "takes phonics, which is the F-word in today's society, at least in the education community," Lyon says. "But phonics is nothing more than a relationship between sound structure and a print structure. Phonics is absolutely essential, non-negotiable. You can't read English without it" (2004). (More phonics findings are discussed under the heading "The Fury over Sounds" below.)

The third big idea—*fluency*—means being able to take the foundational skills of phonemic awareness and phonics and run with them. To be readers, kids need "the rapid application of those print-level skills to text," Lyon says (2004). Shaywitz explains the brain processes that foster fluency this way: "Fluency—reading a word accurately, quickly, smoothly, and with good expression—is acquired by practice, by reading a word over and over again. This is consistent with what we know about neural circuits that are reinforced and strengthened with repetition. A reader must have four or more successful encounters with a word to be able to read it fluently" (2003, 105).

Of the fourth big idea—*vocabulary*—Lyon makes this statement: "If kids don't have vocabulary, they won't understand what the heck they're reading" (2004). This statement may seem ridiculously obvious. Yet direct instruction in words—their connotations and denotations, their usages, their origins— often gets neglected in schools. Shaywitz explains the importance of building vocabulary: "Reading is more than associating letters with sounds. The aspiring reader must build his reading vocabulary so that eventually he can read complex, long, or unfamiliar words" (2003, 103).

Here's how Shaywitz describes the process of amassing a wide and workable store of words:

> The child goes from storing images of individual letters associated with specific sounds to storing larger and larger chunks of printed material—common letters that frequently go together (*-at*, *-gh*, *-th*), larger groups of letters that recur (*-ight*, *-eight*, *-ought*), and, finally, after the child has read many books and successfully decoded thousands of words again and again, he has accumulated a storehouse of entire words. (2003, 104)

Building a big vocabulary depends on the same letter-by-letter processing described above by Adams and Torgesen. Writes Shaywitz, "To acquire a new word for his vocabulary, a child must scrutinize the inner details of the word and not gloss over it. For the most part, analyzing each letter and letter group in a word is the only way an accurate stored representation is formed and the most effective means of having a new written word become a part of the child's working vocabulary" (2003, 106).

But that's not all. The fifth and final big idea—*comprehension*—is clearly the reason for nurturing the other four skills, the very reason we read. Consider this quote: "Good comprehenders link the ideas presented in print to their own experiences." It sounds like it could be a message straight from the mouths of the constructivists. But in fact, it's a quote from the research community, indeed from the very Reid Lyon who is often disparaged in whole-language chat rooms as the "poster boy for phonics," and accused of ignoring or minimizing the importance of meaning in reading instruction. When he talks about comprehension skills, Lyon's words could easily be mistaken for a verbatim passage from the whole-language handbook. "Good comprehenders," he says, "have a knack for summarizing, predicting, and clarifying what they have read, and many are adept at asking themselves guide questions to enhance understanding" (1998, 16).

Research is no Johnny-come-lately in its discovery of the importance of meaning in reading, or the essential link between phonics and comprehension. As long ago as the 1960s, studies were coalescing around the finding that early achievement in decoding aids comprehension *as well as* word recognition. A series of basic research studies published in the decade and a half after *The Great Debate* confirmed this finding. "Essentially," Chall says, "they indicate that word recognition and ability to decode individual words is basic to reading comprehension" (Chall 1983, 27).

The "big ideas in reading" are like a Mobius strip or an M. C. Escher image, where you can't find the beginning or the end because it all flows together seamlessly. "Phonemic awareness is a cause as well as a consequence of literacy acquisition, with each influencing the other as children learn to read and spell," researcher Linnea Ehri has discovered. "The relationship is thought to be reciprocal with cause running in both directions" (1998, 107). The same can be said of phonics and comprehension, phonics and vocabulary, vocabulary and fluency, fluency and comprehension.

While the evidence has converged sufficiently around the five big ideas to give them wide consensus among researchers, other factors are under study as well. For example, Berninger's team is taking a close look at how orthography, morphology, and executive function figure into the dyslexia equation.

In bringing the "big ideas" to the classroom, the teacher's judgment is essential to success. "The teacher has to know how to assess that range of foundational building blocks—phonemic awareness, phonics, fluency, vocabulary, comprehension—and has to assess the program intensity and clarity in terms of teaching those for those kids and then modify, adjust," Lyon says (2004).

5. The Fury over Sounds

Although phonics is only one of the five "big ideas," it has had a lopsided effect on the debate. The sound and fury over phonics has been a kind of perfect storm, sinking the progress of millions of young readers.

The first step in learning phonics, however, is a pre-phonics skill—what has been called an "ear skill" (although we know that the skill actually originates in the brain, rather than the ear itself). The ability to hear the individual sounds (phonemes) that form spoken words—phonemic awareness—is as essential to the young reader as seawater is to a starfish. "Phonological skills influence reading from the start," Shaywitz writes (2003, 145). She cites a study by a group of Florida researchers led by Torgesen that demonstrated the "profound impact" these skills have on a child's later reading. The Florida study found that "children who began first grade with poor phonologic skills (in the lowest 20 percent of their class) were two grade levels below their classmates in a test of word reading in fifth grade" (Shaywitz 2003, 145).

Lyon explains the need for direct, explicit instruction in the sound-symbol structure of printed language like this: "Nature has provided a conundrum here: What is good for the listener—seamless blending of sounds into 'bundles'—is not so good for the beginning reader. Although spoken language is seamless, the beginning reader must detect the seams in speech, unglue the sounds from one another, and learn which sounds (phonemes) go with which letters" (1998, 18). By the end of first grade, children should have just about mastered their basic phonologic skills if they are going to move ahead with reading. "From second grade on," says Shaywitz, "a child's development of these competencies is more a matter of refining and gaining efficiency or automaticity in the phonological skills previously acquired" (2003, 144).

The research record on this is full of hard evidence. When Chall updated *The Great Debate* in 1983, research suggested that direct instruction in phonics is more effective than the indirect phonics approaches used in most classrooms today (if, indeed, phonics is taught at all). "It would seem," Chall wrote, "that many of the characteristics of direct phonics, such as teaching letter-sounds directly, separating the letter-sounds from the words, giving practice in blending the sounds, and so forth are more effective" than procedures that "teach letter sounds indirectly from known sight words by inference and generalization" (43). For disadvantaged and LD children in particular, Chall said, the evidence favors a direct approach (1983).

The National Reading Panel "concluded that the results of a meta-analysis of the results of 66 comparisons from 38 different studies indicated 'solid support for the conclusion that systematic phonics instruction makes a bigger contribution to children's growth in reading than alternative programs providing unsystematic or no phonics instruction'" (Stanovich and Stanovich 2003, 18). In another section of its report, the NRP reported that a meta-analysis of fifty-two studies of phonemic awareness training indicated that "teaching children to manipulate the sounds in language helps them learn to read. . . . Effects of phonemic awareness training on reading lasted well beyond the end of training" (Stanovich and Stanovich 2003, 18).

In the twenty years since Chall, the evidence has continued to multiply. Decades of careful research have shown that revealing the sound-symbol code directly and systematically is what "allows a child to cross the threshold into the world of reading," in Shaywitz's words. "Children can memorize hundreds of words," she says, "but by the time they reach fifth grade, they will come across as many as 10,000 new words during the school year. Relying on memorization simply won't do. To make progress in reading, they must learn how the alphabetic code works. Linking letters to sounds and then sounding out words is the only guarantee of being able to decode the thousands of new words" (2003, 102–3).

Shaywitz explains the indispensability of decoding this way: "The beauty of this process," she says, "is that it allows the reader to decipher and read a word that she has never before encountered. She sees a word and scans all the letters. Do any of the letters fall into a familiar pattern? Do they resemble letter groups—parts of words—that she has stored? If so, she is able to take these letter patterns and connect them to a known pronunciation" (2003, 104).

6. In Spite of Poverty

Research in actual schools has shown over and over that with research-based methods, even kids living in deprivation can learn to read. "A number of longitudinal treatment studies pointed to the same conclusion—reading problems could be prevented, or the severity of their expression reduced to a large extent, with appropriate intervention, even if children came from low-literacy homes," Berninger writes (2006).

One remarkable "living laboratory" study has shown astronomical gains in reading skills for disadvantaged students in Tallahassee, Florida. The scores of the mostly poor and minority kids who attend Hartsfield Elementary School went from grim to great between 1995 to 1999 after the school adopted a research-based approach to reading instruction. At the beginning of the study, 32 percent of first-graders were in the bottom quarter on word-attack and word-identification assessments. Five years later, only 4 percent were in the lowest quartile. First-graders who could read rose from half to over 80 percent. The median percentile in reading achievement for third-graders taking the California Achievement Test rose from 49 to 73 between 1994 and 1999.

The school also saw a shift in staff attitudes, notes Hartsfield Principal Ray King in a report detailing the project. Teachers, he said, had "developed a culture of acceptance of failure" for struggling students, "blaming the home and lack of parental support" (King and Torgesen 2000, 1). Hartsfield, working closely with Torgesen, abandoned its "every-teacher-for-herself" philosophy, putting into place a unified, coordinated reading curriculum that featured schoolwide block scheduling, small-group instruction, and ongoing reading assessments. Early childhood and prekindergarten services were expanded and enhanced.

7. The Myth of "Catching Up"

Everyone has had one of those dreams where you're trying to run, you're straining as hard as you can to move forward, but your legs feel leaden, your feet feel riveted to the ground. You're going nowhere. For kids who fall behind in reading, that nightmare is their everyday reality. Because no matter how the child's teacher may soothe his parents' worries by explaining that kids learn to read at their own pace, that "he'll catch up," studies show that without intensive, research-supported intervention, he won't. "Scientific data show that reading problems are persistent; they do not represent a temporary lag in development," Shaywitz says. "It is wishful thinking to believe there will be a sudden magical improvement. Schools often have a tendency to want to wait" (2003, 128).

Even for a child who is not dyslexic but who fails to learn to read along with her classmates, catching up is a chimera. For each week during which reading eludes her, the other kids are building fluency, vocabulary, and comprehension skills. In a study of reading disabilities in 10,000 children, Gilbert B. Schiffman found that of kids diagnosed in grades one or two, about 80 percent were brought up to grade level. But the success rate fell off sharply after that. Only about 45 percent of kids who were not diagnosed until grades 3 or 4 caught up to their peers. And kids whose disability was not identified until grade 5, 6, or 7 had only a 10 percent to 15 percent chance of achieving grade-level reading skills (Berninger, Thalberg, DeBruyn, and Smith 1987).

The only hope for children with reading problems is prevention and early intervention. The "wait-to-fail" model, which has been the traditional approach in U.S. schools, has had devastating consequences, emotionally and academically, for millions of children. "If a child is dyslexic early on in school, that child will continue to experience reading problems *unless he is provided with a scientifically based, proven intervention*" (Shaywitz 2003, 34, italics added). For children who struggle, sitting them in front of a book for fifteen minutes of SSR (silent sustained reading) is an exercise in futility. Research shows that instead, they need guided oral reading—in a safe environment—and direct instruction in vocabulary and comprehension skills.

As Adams reports, research "demonstrates that, with the exception of no more than 1 percent to 3 percent of children, reading disability can be prevented through well-designed early instruction. . . . [S]uch instruction must include attention to phonics, and is most effective when it includes explicit, systematic instruction on the alphabetic principle, including phonemic awareness and on the spelling-sound patterns and conventions of English, as well as an active emphasis on practicing and using that knowledge both in isolation and in the context of meaningful reading and writing" (1998, 86).

8. Support for Three Tiers

"Reading failure is one of a small group of public health problems that we have the ability to detect reliably early on, treat effectively, and even perhaps prevent," Shaywitz writes. "We must ensure that each child who is not learning to read in the first year or so of school is identified and treated. It is now possible to protect children against reading failure, but in order to do so, such children must first be identified. The earlier the diagnosis is made, the better the results" (2003, 141).

The three-tier model, first introduced by Gerald Caplan and Henry Grunebaum of Harvard Medical School back in 1967, is being touted by a growing cadre of experts as the best way to prevent reading problems for most kids and to intervene quickly and effectively for those who fail to respond to well-designed instruction. Berninger gives a quick run-down of the focus for each tier: Tier 1—"screening for early intervention"; Tier 2—"ongoing progress monitoring and supplementary intervention throughout school"; Tier 3—"differential diagnosis and specialized treatment for those with persisting, biologically based specific learning disabilities" (2006).

The National Association of School Psychologists recommended the three-tier model to Congress in its latest rewriting of the IDEA legislation. "While recognizing that no single model of identification of learning disabilities will address all philosophies and concerns, the recommended Three-Tiered Model reflects best practices in assessment and data-based decision-making," NASP asserted (2003).

To head off problems before they begin, you have to start early. "Many experts recommend that large-scale screening for phonologic difficulties be carried out during the second semester of kindergarten, when the child is about five and a half or even six years old," Shaywitz says. "At this point all the children have been exposed to at least one semester of formal schooling and should have developed some degree of phonologic ability" (2003, 143).

Because research has shown that "phonemic awareness has the strongest relationship to later reading," Shaywitz continues, "most tests focus on this level of awareness" (2003, 143). She says, "The most helpful tests include three kinds of measures: sound comparison, segmentation, and blending" (144).

A body of research is building that backs up the tiered approach. One example is a statewide pilot project tested at eighteen schools in Washington State. The Student Responsive Delivery System is a Tier 2 model sponsored by the state office of public instruction, the Washington State Association of School Psychologists, and the Washington State Speech and Hearing Association. The model has reaped impressive gains, based on findings from the

1998–1999 school year. Of the 215 students who participated in the collaborative problem-solving process, 138 students (64 percent) needed no further intervention. Their academic and/or behavioral troubles were resolved. The number of students who needed a full-blown assessment for special ed was axed by a staggering 73 percent across the pilot sites. Ultimately, only twenty-eight students (13 percent) were placed in special ed.

"Today," Shaywitz says, "it is possible to reliably identify boys and girls at high risk for dyslexia *before* they fall behind" (2003, 142). In the following chapter, we take readers to a school district that is doing just that, using the three-tier model as a framework and achieving remarkable results with a student population that is typically on the bottom rung of reading achievement.

9. Lagging Behind in the Resource Room

A number of studies have found that the "resource room"—the small-group pull-out model for special ed used in most schools—is, at best, effective only in preventing further slippage relative to the child's classmates. Berninger is blunt. "Special education for students with learning disabilities," she says, "has not been effective."

The instruction provided in most resource rooms is not intensive enough or powerful enough to bring the child up to parity with his or her peers. The Connecticut study found that the special help children were receiving "might best be described as a Band-aid approach to a gushing wound," Shaywitz says. "In general we found that children received help for very limited periods of time, often from well-meaning but untrained teachers and with methods that did not reflect state-of-the-art, evidence-based instructional strategies" (2003, 35).

One revealing study led by Sharon Vaughn of the University of Texas at Austin found that students in a large, southeastern district were virtually treading water in their resource rooms. The reading scores of eighty-plus elementary students across fourteen pull-outs actually *skidded downward* from fall to spring—from a mean of 15.56 on the Stanford Achievement Test at the beginning of the year to 14.19 at the end (Vaughn, Moody, and Schumm 1998). The researchers observed pull-out classes with as many as fifteen students who were getting mainly whole-group instruction based primarily on the whole-language philosophy. Direct, targeted, individualized teaching was slim to none. In fact, the resource-room experience of these special-ed kids—94 percent LD—was barely distinguishable from the regular classroom experience. "We think that the findings of this study reveal a series of broken promises," Vaughn and fellow researchers Sally Moody and Jeanne Schumm concluded. "The most obvious is the broken promise to the student and the parent that an individualized reading program will be provided to each student to meet their specific needs" (1998, 222).

10. Intensive Intervention for LD Kids

Research has found that children on the far end of the continuum of reading disability—those with biologically based disorders—need more time, more intensity, and more support. Barbara Foorman and Torgesen say,

> The components of effective reading instruction are the same whether the focus is prevention or intervention: phonemic awareness and phonemic decoding skills, fluency in word recognition and text processing, construction of meaning, vocabulary, spelling, and writing. Findings from evidence-based research show dramatic reductions in the incidence of reading failure when explicit instruction in these components is provided by the classroom teacher. To address the needs of children most at risk of reading failure, the same instructional components are relevant but they need to be made more explicit and comprehensive, more intensive, and more supportive in small-group or one-on-one formats. (2001, 203)

"MOVING SCIENCE TO HUMAN BEINGS"

"How do we fill in the informational lacuna such that we can actually move science to human beings, science to policy, science to practice?" Lyon wonders.

> The toughest challenge we have is in moving the science to the development of teachers and their preparation, such that what they learn is actually objective and is based upon converging evidence rather than philosophies, belief systems, or appeals to authority. We need to get the information to teachers who have been, in a sense, propagandized into these very broad and general and non-evidentiary kinds of approaches that they use in teaching reading—absolute failures in terms of our scientific tests vis-à-vis their effectiveness. (2004)

Lyon will aim to do just that in his new position as senior vice president of research and evaluation for Best Associates, which underwrites start-up companies, including education ventures. In May 2005, Lyon announced that he and his partners are launching a teacher education initiative to develop a national college of education.

GOOD BOOKS ON READING: A MUST-READ LIST ON SCIENCE-BASED INSTRUCTION

For educators and parents who want to immerse themselves in reading research without drowning in jargon and verbosity, we recommend the six publications below. Taken as a whole, they will give you a comprehensive overview of reading research. Several of them summarize and synthesize decades of research—a practical way to digest critical information from thousands of articles, books, and reports.

1. *Preventing Reading Difficulties in Young Children* (1998)

The National Research Council's seminal report (Snow, Burns, and Griffin 1998), in tandem with the next book on the list by the National Reading Panel, has been called a "consensus" report because it pulls from a broad base of thinking, expertise, and research on reading. Written by the Committee on the Prevention of Reading Difficulties in Young Children, chaired by Catherine Snow of Harvard's Graduate School of Education, the book draws upon the expertise of psychologists, neurobiologists, and educators to establish clear recommendations for guiding all children toward a lifetime of literacy. Quotes on the book's back cover include one from the *New York Times*, calling it the book that "could serve as a road map to national standards." *Newsday* said it "tackles some of the most explosive issues in education." It caused the *Boston Globe* to declare, "The contentious, decades-long debate over how to teach reading is over."

2. *Teaching Children to Read* (2000)

Also available in summary format, this report of the National Reading Panel is what Sally Shaywitz of Yale calls the first "evidence-based" guide to what works in teaching children to read. "It is an outgrowth of a grassroots concern that while a substantial number of children were failing to learn to read, little was available to help parents and teachers make important choices among different approaches to reading instruction," she says (2003, 174). In 1997, Congress directed the creation of the panel of experts and charged them with doing an objective, comprehensive review of the existing research on reading. The book, says Shaywitz, "provides a road map to guide parents and teachers to the most effective, scientifically proven methods for teaching reading. Now in education, as in medicine, we can look to scientific evidence as the basis for choosing a treatment. Before selecting a reading program, parents and teachers can and must ask, 'What is the evidence of its efficacy?'" (2003, 175).

3. *Beginning to Read* (1990)

This classic work by Marilyn Jager Adams is admittedly a pretty intense read in places. But it's essential for anyone who's looking for answers to the big questions in literacy acquisition. Here's how the publisher bills the book on the back cover:

> *Beginning to Read* reconciles the debate that has divided theorists for decades over the "right" way to help children learn to read. Drawing on a rich array of research on the nature and development of reading proficiency, Adams shows educators that they need not remain trapped in the phonics versus teaching-for-meaning dilemma. She proposes that phonics can work together with the whole-language approach to teaching reading and provides an integrated treatment of the knowledge and process involved in skillful reading, the issues surrounding their acquisition, and the implications for reading instruction. (1990b)

Stahl, Osborn, and Lehr have compressed Adams's book into a more digestible, less technical summary published by the Center for the Study of Reading, Champaign, University of Illinois, 1990.

4. *Using Research and Reason in Education* (2003)

This forty-two-page booklet by Paula J. Stanovich and Keith E. Stanovich of the University of Toronto offers a pithy explanation of the basics of distinguishing science from pseudoscience. Although the booklet doesn't focus on reading per se, the authors offer examples from the reading controversy to illustrate their points. For teachers who are uncomfortable with—or confused about—how scientific method meshes with educational methodology, this booklet can help to clarify these connections. Copies of the booklet can be ordered from the National Institute for Literacy at EdPubs, P. O. Box 1398, Jessup, MD 20794-1398. Call 800-228-8813 or email edpubs@inet.ed.gov.

5. *Overcoming Dyslexia* (2003)

Shaywitz's masterpiece on reading disabilities is simply the best explanation available on the brain differences that cause them and the research-based strategies for preventing and treating them. Shaywitz, a neuroscientist and professor of pediatrics at the Yale Center for the Study of Learning and Attention, is a giant of the reading-research community. She has pulled together her decades of pioneering work in this book that is not only full of science, but also of passion. As Daniel Federman of Harvard Medical School aptly observes on the book jacket, "In this gem of a book, Dr. Sally Shaywitz uses her voice, her images, her brain—and, yes, her heart—to shine a piercing and clarifying light on what we so inadequately call 'dyslexia.' What is more, she shows how almost everyone can overcome it."

6. *Straight Talk about Reading* (1999)

This practical book is aimed at parents of kids in kindergarten through third grade. Written by Susan Hall, an activist who is the parent of a dyslexic child, and Louisa Cook Moats, a prominent reading expert, this appealing book with the bright yellow cover provides easily digestible information on how kids learn to read, along with useful tips for moms and dads who want to take "a proactive stance" in their child's education. The book promises to provide background on the differences between whole language and phonics approaches; ways to determine if your child's teacher is using effective teaching practices; benchmark lists to see whether your child is "on track"; a list of warning signs for reading difficulty; and lists of recommended books scaled by reading difficulty.

"TEACHERS ARE HUNGRY FOR INFORMATION ABOUT THE BRAIN"

Grim as they were, the ghettos and barrios of America looked better than the jungles of wartime Vietnam to a lot of university students in the early 1970s. Under a federal program aimed at filling a desperate shortage of inner-city teachers, young men and women could opt to serve their country in the 'hood.

One who answered the call was Virginia Berninger. Just out of college and ready for a stint in the real world before heading back to academia as a graduate student, Berninger spent a year teaching fifty African American and Puerto Rican third-graders in the heart of Philadelphia—no bombs, no napalm, but a jungle just the same.

"We had police escorts because of the gangs in the streets," she says, recalling the rawness of the children's lives with fresh force some three decades later. "I had kids who didn't return from vacation because they were killed or they died of encephalitis, things like that. It was a real eye-opener."

Evenings, she took classes at Temple University, where she delved into the psychology of reading—a natural for a psychology major who'd had a lifelong fascination with how the brain processes the written word and why some children struggle to learn. Berninger's graduate education at the Johns Hopkins University was in experimental psychology, focusing on the three areas she thought "held the clue to figuring out what to do with learning disabilities"—cognitive psychology, psychobiology, and psycholinguistics. Her postdoctoral work took her to Boston Children's Hospital, where she taught with a group of physicians from all over the country about child development and learning disabilities and worked in clinics serving children with developmental and learning disorders.

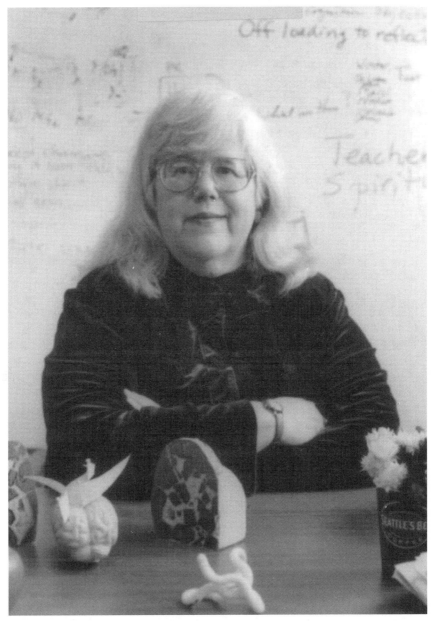

Virginia Berninger

Now a widely published professor in the University of Washington College of Education School Psychology Program and director of the UW Multidisciplinary Learning Disabilities Center, Berninger designs and oversees cutting-edge research on the brain-based learning disorders and strategies for addressing learning differences. The center, one of several such centers housed at universities around the nation (including Yale and Georgetown), is engaged in research on brain imaging, as well as genetic clues to learning disabilities. The UW brain imaging team, headed by Todd Richards and Elizabeth Aylward, has discovered, for example, that dyslexic children differ from good readers in brain activation associated with several language tasks, but these differences disappear after instructional intervention.

Sitting in her office among teetering paper towers of research reports and scholarly journals, Berninger shares a sampling of her knowledge and experience.

Q: Why is it important for teachers to study the brain?

BERNINGER: I find that teachers are hungry for information about the brain. Yet there's so much bogus information out there. It's very easy to be naïve—to not be a critical consumer of what's out there. There are a lot of people who are capitalizing on this gap in teachers' knowledge. It also concerns me because teachers are expected to help kids learn and develop, and the major organ for that is the brain. Yet they are given no training for this in their teacher education programs. Neuroscience has been around for about 150 years, and we're getting to the point where there are certain general principles that are givens—a body of shared knowledge. Not that we fully understand the brain by a long shot. But if you don't understand these principles, you're going to remain a naïve consumer of this information.

Q: What is the connection between reading and writing difficulties?

BERNINGER: Kids with reading problems generally also have writing problems. Writing disabilities are less understood, even, than reading disabilities. One of the first grants I got was looking at individual differences among children in their abilities to write letters, words, sentences, and texts. I was looking for the early developmental origin of writing problems, instead of waiting until the upper elementary or middle school years after years of chronic failure. We think we found it: It's handwriting and it's spelling. And, more importantly, it's handwriting "automaticity"—how automatically the student can make those letters so they're not drawing them. It needs to be automatic so you're not using valuable mental resources for making the letters, and you have more room to think about what you want to say and how you're going to say it. Spelling is a way of representing the sound system of spoken language. So children who have trouble with that sound system, with those phonemes and translating or mapping those phonemes onto letters, are the ones who have the spelling difficulty. Most schools use whole language and journal writing, where there isn't a lot of explicit instruction and attention to transcription. I think the whole-language approach may have created a lot of writing disabled kids—kids who are curriculum casualties, not biologically based writing casualties.

Q: But curriculum design doesn't hold all the answers, does it?

BERNINGER: We knew it wasn't totally curriculum because, let's be honest, there are an awful lot of kids out there who, even with whole language, do pretty well. So our study also looked at writing from a neurodevelopmental point of view: What brain processes were causing the handwriting and the spelling to break down? Although some children are at risk because of biological risk factors—genes, brain wiring—it doesn't mean they can't learn. It's just that for them, it really matters what kind of instruction they get. It needs to be explicit. This doesn't mean you have to drill them to death. It means you have to make it really clear and obvious to them. You have to take all these skills and break them down into little pieces and help them learn all the processes.

Q: So schools need to look at curriculum first?

BERNINGER: When we design intervention plans, we should start by assessing the curriculum, not the child. We need to ask, what are the necessary instructional components that need to be in place? Let's not blame the teachers. Let's not blame the families. Some people still think LD kids are from dysfunctional families and have a motivational problem. That's not the case. These kids don't come from dysfunctional families any more than anyone else. So let's look in the classroom, let's see what's been tried, and see if we can help the school tweak it, add some things, delete some things, modify some things.

Q: How does the teacher know whether her approach is working on an individual basis—whether each child is making sufficient gains?

BERNINGER: It's got to be an integrated assessment-intervention approach. You need to build in daily progress monitoring—a way for the child to get a little sense of progress. You need to quickly get the kids to feel like, "I can do it"—to feel like they're readers and writers—because motivation is such an important part. You need to set goals and monitor progress weekly, monthly, and twice a year using a variety of modes of assessment. A lot of teachers just aren't comfortable with the assessment role, and they don't do it. That's why they don't know that some kids aren't making it. If a kid sits there smiling or is socially appropriate or says cute things, the teacher just doesn't realize there's a problem.

Q: What strategies have you developed that help ensure that all kinds of learners grasp reading in the early years?

BERNINGER: We have found that kids' word recognition gets better when they work on both the alphabetic principle and comprehension—that you really need to teach all of it. We've tried to integrate the best of the skills approach with the best of whole language.

Q: Can you really blend whole language with direct instruction in sound-letter patterns?

BERNINGER: If I were helping schools evolve, I would have tracks where you cover the same kind of material with all kids in an intellectually engaging way, but some kids get more explicit instruction. Some kids need that explicitness; others can figure it out on their own.

Q: Have schools in general made progress in working with LD kids?

BERNINGER: In the '70s most teacher education programs had very little formal instruction on how to teach reading. I think that's changed in some places, but it hasn't changed everywhere. I don't want to fault any one group. I just think as a nation, we still have not come to terms with the fact that there are both biologically based and culturally based learning differences. We're not adequately preparing teachers in a practical sense for what they can do, day to day, in their classroom to deal with this diversity.

"THE WHOLE LANGUAGE-PHONICS DICHOTOMY IS A TERRIBLE DICHOTOMY"

When Edward Kame'enui walked to the podium at the White House, he was nearing the apex of a journey that had started in obscurity some thirty years earlier. No one, least of all Kame'enui himself, could have predicted that his work with a motley crew of troubled kids in the 1970s would culminate in an address to a polished audience at the White House Conference on Preparing Tomorrow's Teachers in 2004. In the decades between, the University of Oregon professor and researcher had become a standard-bearer in the movement to teach reading in a direct, systematic way—a movement that, after years of brutal bashing and battering by opposing forces, is finally taking its place at the table of educational respectability.

So there he was at the center of power and policymaking in Washington, D.C., making his case for the need to transform reading instruction in schools all across America. As the then-director of the UO Institute for the Develop-

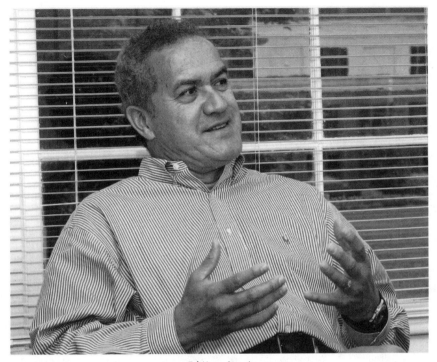

Ed Kame'enui

ment of Educational Achievement, Kame'enui led a team of reading research-ers that drew notoriety—and often bitter controversy—as champions of direct instruction. Kame'enui spoke that day with passionate eloquence, quoting such thinkers as Harold Bloom, Jonathan Kozol, Horace Mann, and Mark Twain in an in-kind demonstration of the fruits of literacy.

As he built his argument for research-based teaching, he cast a stern indict-ment on the idea that reading is "natural" and that, therefore, explicit teach-ing is unnecessary. If children are "left to the winds of chance and the vagaries of incidental learning," most can never hope to taste the "beguiling soliloquies of Shakespeare" or tackle a scientific text with success, Kame'e-nui told the audience of educators and policymakers. "Reading the words matters, and reading the right words matters even more," he said, and then offered this typically cogent remark from American literary icon Mark Twain: "The difference between the almost right word and the right word is really a large matter—'tis the difference between the lightning bug and the lightning."

Kame'enui wrapped up his speech with a poetic reference to Polynesian folklore. He told his audience that according to tradition, the Hawaiian greeting "aloha" means "the lighted breath without end." He left them with the suggestion that reading is just that—"truly the lighted breath without end."

Just a year after the Hawaii native and former Purdue University professor spoke those words, Kame'enui was heading back to Washington, D.C., this time as the nation's first commissioner for special education research. After nearly two decades at the UO, he left in 2005 to lead the National Center for Special Education Research, a congressionally created office within the U.S. Education Department's Institute of Education Sciences in Washington, D.C.

Q: Why have you chosen to focus so much of your work on early reading skills when your background is in special education? How are the two related?

KAME'ENUI: In the 1970s, I taught for five years at a residential treatment center in Wisconsin for children with serious emotional problems. I had kids from eight years old to eighteen. I realized I could manage kids—I could manage their behavior—but I didn't know what to do with the instruction. I tried different programs, but they weren't very good. At that time, special ed was the only discipline within education that focused on the architecture of information, the design of instruction. If you go to the research literature in experimental psychology, you find a whole body of literature on designing instruction. In special ed, I could focus on my interest in the architecture—how to communicate ideas, how to deliver information, how to structure the full range of content to teach kids.

Q: Was it your sense that some of those emotional and behavioral problems were related to untreated learning disabilities?

KAME'ENUI: Directly. The kids I had, with the exception of maybe two kids in five years, had serious academic problems. When a task was too hard, they'd be in your face because they didn't know how to do it. But once you structured it and eased them into the complexity, they had success and they were different. I realized that the way to change behavior was to make sure kids were successful academically.

Q: What does the typical reading program look like today?

KAME'ENUI: The typical program is a commercial program that tries to accommodate most kids—80 percent, maybe fewer. Its architecture is horizontal, not vertical. It tries to cover a lot of information, a lot of topics, so it can't go very deep on any one topic. It typically offers two or three examples, and models those examples once or twice. It rarely offers sufficient practice, rarely offers sufficient scaffolding, rarely offers explicit teacher support. It rarely provides a systematic, cumulative review.

Q: Would you say the typical reading program in America is geared for kids from the educated middle class?

KAME′ENUI: Sure. Absolutely. Publishers recognize that this has to change. You can't reach all kids with one undifferentiated program. One size doesn't fit all.

Q: What needs to happen to break down the barriers between whole language and phonics advocates?

KAME′ENUI: We so often want to reduce these things to black and white, and it's just not that simple. The whole-language–phonics dichotomy to me is really a terrible dichotomy. It's useless because it fails to capture the complexity of the English language and the alphabetic writing system. I don't agree that the whole-language movement is impervious to research. I think they are very tuned in, but to their own particular kind of research. What that invokes is a whole set of questions around what is research and what is the nature of science. They would argue that their research just taps a different form of inquiry, one that isn't anchored to causal research designs—quasi-experimental or experimental designs—but is more qualitative. The fundamental problem with the whole-language approach is that it assumes the learner can take in linguistic cues in a way that is not consistent with what we know about how kids learn. Kids simply don't pick up print and its meanings incidentally. The whole-language assumption is that if you just sample enough of the print, you'll understand the alphabetic writing system. That's not the case. But there are some pieces of whole language that are very important. We have gotten into dichotomies that just simply are vulgar— dichotomies that don't permit us to really think seriously about the problem, that have led us off course.

Q: But some kids *can* take a few linguistic cues and take off without direct instruction.

KAME′ENUI: When I was on the Committee on the Prevention of Reading Difficulties in Young Children, that was one of the questions: Doesn't reading come naturally? It appears that reading does come naturally for maybe 5 percent of kids—kids who somehow intuit the writing system. They're able to make the connection between the sounds they're hearing and the print on the page. But that leaves 95 percent who need some kind of intentional arrangement of the environment. Language comes naturally, but not the writing system.

Q: You emphasize what you call the "essential linkage" of assessment and

instruction in a kind of feedback loop. How is assessment used in the
typical school?

KAME′ENUI: In a typical school, children are assessed maybe once a
year. The kind of assessment that gets the most play in the newspaper is
outcome assessment at the end of the year—where are our kids at the
end of third grade? How are our kids doing on the statewide tests? That
kind of assessment tells me, as a teacher, whether my kids are at benchmark, but it's not very useful for guiding instruction day to day. The
kind of assessment I think is absolutely critical is ongoing progress
monitoring and screening. We want to identify kids early on, and we
want to monitor their performance every two weeks if we can. And we
want to do it in a way that is absolutely most efficient. That means that
you can't spend a lot of time.

Q: And DIBELS—the Dynamic Indicators of Basic Early Literacy—
developed here at UO would fit the bill?

KAME′ENUI: DIBELS is one kind of measurement system, but there are
others that take very quick samples of children's reading behavior and
have enough predictive power to tell us about the future. In the absence
of that, I don't know how you would adjust instruction. Right now,
teachers are using portfolio assessment and their own hunches. The predictive power of those things is marginal, at best.

Q: A lot of educators feel that a science-based approach is not sufficiently
humanistic.

KAME′ENUI: That's right. I worry that too many educators see this as
humanistic versus non-humanistic. It's the dichotomies again. The system is too complex for dichotomies.

Q: What was the impact of the National Research Council's 1998 report,
Preventing Reading Difficulties in Young Children, on public policy and
classroom practice? As a member of the committee that compiled the
report, were you satisfied with its impact?

KAME′ENUI: At the time, it was clearly significant because the report
was sponsored by the National Academy of Sciences. NAS is a unique,
independent entity that doesn't take on a scientific issue unless it knows
there is evidence to resolve the problem. It was a significant statement
in the field of education: Look, whether you like it or not, we have the
research to adjudicate these issues. We don't have to get into serious
argumentation with each other and point fingers and get rancorous. Let's
look at the scientific evidence. It also set the stage for the National Reading Panel. The NRP report is, to me, the most significant evidence
because it is a quantitative meta-analysis.

Q: The NRP was criticized for having too many experts from disciplines like psychology, pediatrics, and neurology versus education. Have you run into that criticism?

KAME'ENUI: Sure. Many people don't understand that reading is a truly interdisciplinary topic. That's why medicine is involved, that's why pediatric neurologists are involved, that's why experimental psychologists are involved. I think we've lost sight of the fact that learning happens in the brain. Psychologists deal with the question, How do you get information into memory so you retain it? How do you lay it down so that it can be recalled time and time again, instantly? And how do we get kids to the point where they're very fast with it? Even the International Reading Association will recognize that reading is interdisciplinary.

Q: What other criticisms did you run into?

KAME'ENUI: Many people also criticized the NRP report because it didn't capture all of the research. Educational research is in what Thomas Kuhn would call a "pre-paradigmatic" phase, where we don't have a solid paradigm of inquiry. We don't have a science with first-order learning principles—definitions of the most basic constructs, such as learning, that are critical to our field. For example, if you asked educators to define learning, ten educators would give you ten responses. As a result, all evidence appears to be equal—your research versus my research, your opinion versus my opinion. Anything goes. That's not the case in the hard sciences. Physics and chemistry have first-order principles. If you violate those principles, people just don't pay attention to you. The criticism of the NRP report is not about the report, it's about the immaturity of our science. The report was critical because it applied the most rigorous, quantitative standards we have to the science and it says, "Look, if you apply these standards, you'll get these results." Of the 100,000 studies done since 1966, only a handful, maybe 2 percent, met the NRP benchmark for standards. That's terrible. We have to learn how to do better science.

"THIS IS A REAL CONVERGENCE AMONG RESEARCHERS"

It was a "lucky accident" that propelled Roland Good into his life's work. It was the early 1970s. Guys his age were sweating out the draft and, when the lottery was instituted, praying for a lucky number. While antiwar protests raged on college campuses across the United States, thousands of young men were shipping out to Vietnam. Good was among a select few who had been granted conscientious-objector status—a designation that kept him out of the jungle, but not out of fulfilling an obligation to the country. He was "drafted" to serve at the School of Hope in Williamsport, Pennsylvania, as a teacher's aide for intellectually disabled youths. "I had been really looking for what I wanted to do with my life," Good remembers. "Working with children made my eyes sparkle."

As he talks about his career as a teacher, a school psychologist, and, these days, a prominent researcher in the field of reading disability, Good seems in danger of falling off the swivel chair that barely contains his tall frame, so expansive are his gestures, so impassioned is his delivery. His eyes widen with boyish exuberance as he describes the ongoing, sixteen-year development of the innovative assessment tool DIBELS (Dynamic Indicators of Basic Early Literacy Skills)—a team effort that he leads. When asked who's using DIBELS these days, he says, "Man, a whole lot of people." Doing some quick mental math, he reports that something like 5,000 schools in forty-five states have adopted the DIBELS Data System, impacting one million students. Canadian and overseas American schools are using DIBELS, too. There's a version in Spanish, a version in French, and discussions are underway to extend it into other languages. "We would like to see it become really very big," Good says.

Listening to the energy in his voice, you might get the idea that Good stands to make money on this product. But that would be a misreading of his enthusiasm. "We *give* it away," he says. By simply going to the DIBELS website at http://dibels.uoregon.edu anyone can download the tool for free and make unlimited copies for educational use. "If you're a school without a lot of resources and you want a powerful, effective tool, DIBELS is there for you," Good notes. "The price is right."

Good radiates a playfulness that might explain, in part, his attraction to working with kids. His erudite discussion of reading research is peppered with the kind of goofy humor that appeals to a lot of adolescents. Explaining, for instance, that the acronym "DIBELS" sticks in people's minds because it has a clever ring to it, he gets an obvious kick out of tossing off a few DIBELS puns to demonstrate: "You can go dibbling," he offers, and, "You can dabble in dibbles." But his humor has a serious subtext. It's not enough to become a whiz at administering DIBELS, he tells teachers. The assessments with the funny name are useless unless they're followed up by effective interventions targeted at the child's specific learning needs.

Q: Your career path took you from special ed to school psychology to your current work in prevention of reading disability. How did you arrive at your focus on reading?

GOOD: I had always felt that reading changed lives for children. When I started practicing as a school psychologist in Erie, Pennsylvania, I found that when children are referred and placed into special ed, it's typically about reading difficulties. But there was this gaping hole in our knowledge base and in our assessment tools for kindergarten and early first grade. We couldn't identify a reading problem with confidence, with accuracy, with reliability, until second or third grade. That was a huge tension for me, professionally. I could see children struggling. I could see problems developing very early. Second or third grade was too late for me to be involved with the prevention of those problems.

Q: You're always playing catch-up.

GOOD: That's exactly right. I wanted to work with kids early, in kindergarten and first grade, to identify concerns, to track progress, to target prevention efforts in a more focused manner. I'm not sure we should identify reading disability in kindergarten, but I think we *should* identify a target of opportunity for teaching and thereby prevent a disability later on.

Q: What do you mean by "target of opportunity"?

GOOD: We now have a pretty good idea of how children learn to read. First, they learn about the sound structure of words. That's the phonological awareness piece. Second, they learn about how letters represent those sounds and go together to form words. That's the alphabetic principle—the phonics—piece. Then they put that all together doing the real thing—reading real words in connected text. Next, they move toward automaticity, and that's Step Three—accuracy and fluency with connected text. Throughout this whole process, we're building vocabulary—Step Four—toward an eventual goal of reading comprehension—Step Five. These are all teachable skills. If a child is struggling with the initial step—learning the sounds in words—that's a target of opportunity. If we can target that skill and if we can teach it, we have the possibility to prevent a serious reading problem later on. For many years, the kindergarten curricula did not teach phonological awareness and did not teach an understanding that words are made up of sounds. That's an opportunity for us, systemically, to change what we teach and what we focus on.

Q: Do you see movement in the field of education toward more acceptance of research and of data-driven decision making?

GOOD: I see huge movement. I see unbelievable movement. If you were to ask me ten years ago to predict where we would be today in that regard, I wouldn't have predicted we'd be anywhere near where we are. But we're still at a point of evolution.

Q: Data are not new phenomena in schools. The shift is in how data are used, right?

GOOD: What's new is using data in a research-based manner to inform our instruction—to really build what we're doing based upon those data.

Q: How is DIBELS different from other assessment systems for early reading indicators?

GOOD: One is a very direct alignment between what DIBELS assesses and the core components of the "big ideas" of early reading—phonemic awareness, phonics, fluency, vocabulary, and comprehension. These are the core components identified by the NRP, but they didn't magically appear with the NRP report. It's not just the panel saying this—this is a real convergence among researchers, among many experts and multiple perspectives over the past thirty years. It's not a coincidence. The exciting thing is how mammoth a convergence this is. In the old days, it was this research group versus that research group. Now there's a sense of all the groups agreeing on the big ideas and moving toward a common agenda.

Q: What else distinguishes DIBELS?

GOOD: Another piece is how incredibly brief the assessments are. We try to measure each of the core components in one minute. In that one minute, we try to get the child to actually demonstrate the goal behavior we want to see. So it's not multiple choice or true/false or fill-in-the-blank. If I want to know how they read connected text, I ask them to read connected text. A teacher who does this one-to-one with a child will get a huge sample of their behavior.

Q: How can you glean so much from a single minute?

GOOD: It requires a very well-designed minute. Our team has been researching and developing DIBELS now for sixteen years. Some member of our research team has probably agonized for a year over some small detail of that minute. However, there is some unreliability around any one-minute measure—was this a bad minute for the student? Did the student have a stomach ache, or was there a fight at home the night before? But the beauty of the DIBELS assessments is that they are not only fast but repeatable. For each of the measures, we have around thirty alternate forms—different ways to assess the same thing. That frees us from the shackle of a single administration of a test—a result that can be compromised if a child is having a bad day. When I test on a repeated basis, I can look for a *pattern* of performance over multiple days under multiple conditions. If the child is consistently in a danger zone, I can be extremely confident that I'm making a good decision about that child.

Q: If assessment is only half of the formula, how do you get across to schools the necessity of doing the other half—the intervention—with integrity?

GOOD: DIBELS can play a remarkable role in that discussion. DIBELS takes a position in a rather unapologetic way: This child has a deficit in phonological awareness. That's not sugar-coated information. A lot of people have asked, "Couldn't you say the child is 'developing' phonological awareness, or something more positive-sounding?" No, they don't have the skill. Almost with the next breath, teachers want to know, "Well, what should I do about it?" The Oregon Curriculum Review Panel and the Oregon Reading First Center have conducted an exhaustive review of intervention programs that target the core components of early literacy. So if DIBELS shows a deficit in, say, the alphabetic principle, a teacher can go to http://reading.uoregon.edu/curricula/or_rfc_review.php and discover, "Gee, Reading Mastery is rated really high, Read Well is rated really high, Voyager Passport is rated really high."

Q: How do you explain the fourth-grade reading slump?

GOOD: In early reading skills, children can take one of two pathways. They can learn words visually, as whole words, and memorize them. Or they can learn the alphabetic principle and how the mechanism works—learn letter sounds and how those sounds form words. If you're learning whole words visually, it looks great at first, but then you crash and burn when you start running into multisyllabic words. A powerful strategy for figuring out a multisyllabic word is to read it syllable by syllable. To do that, you need to have the alphabetic principle. So a child who looks on track, but doesn't have the alphabetic principle, may hit a barrier to their continued reading progress at about third or fourth grade.

5

Before Kids Fail: The Three Tiers of Prevention

There is the very sobering fact obtained in several longitudinal studies that children who are poor readers at the end of first grade almost never acquire average-level reading skills by the end of elementary school.

—Joseph Torgesen
Journal of School Psychology (40, no. 1)

The multi-tiered model ensures that students with learning problems receive supports in general education in a timely manner.

—National Association of School Psychologists
May 2003

Early identification is important because the brain is much more plastic in younger children and potentially more malleable for the rerouting of neural circuits.

—Sally Shaywitz
Overcoming Dyslexia (2003)

One summer evening, Carl Cole was standing in line at the local *taqueria*, a little bit impatient. It was Taco Tuesday at Burrito Amigos—two tacos, two bucks—and he was thinking deeply about the quick-and-cheap meal that was about to quiet the rumbling in his stomach when someone behind him piped up. "Hey, Carl," said a familiar female voice. "How's my favorite special-ed director?"

In that serendipitous moment, the prospects of hundreds of young children suddenly took an upward trajectory. The voice belonged to Cole's longtime acquaintance Deborah Simmons, a University of Oregon professor and researcher (now at Texas A&M) specializing in reading instruction. And just then, Cole's school district was on the cusp of change. He was spearheading a search for strategies to stem an epidemic of special-ed referrals in Bethel.

"Hey, Deb," Carl responded. "Do you want to come out and meet with our administrators?" And so the Bethel Reading Project was seeded.

KIDS ON THE FRINGES

If you drive out to Oregon's Bethel School District, be sure to take along an up-to-date map. The AAA road atlas that's been knocking around your backseat for a few years won't help you much. That's because out here on the northwest fringe of Eugene, low-rent apartments and rows of tract homes are gobbling up pastures and grasslands as fast as a herd of hungry goats. The road you're looking for very likely didn't exist back when your dog-eared atlas was crisp and unsmudged.

Bethel is not so much a suburb of Eugene as a growth spurt. Although it's not far away in miles, it seems unconnected to UO's elm-shaded campus, where students in cargo pants and flip-flops scribble notes in picturesque brick buildings and, after classes, eat pad Thai noodles in laid-back bistros. The main route to the school district offices is an industrial and commercial strip where people shop for RVs and backhoes. Now and then an old barn of dusty mien and rusty hinge sits as though waiting for the bulldozer in its future.

Cole doesn't try to put a pretty face on the place. "If you drove down Highway 99 to get here, you saw the transient hotels and homeless shelters," he tells us on our first visit.

Not surprisingly, most of the children who go to school here are poor. Many of them are immigrants from Mexico or Russia. Mobility is high, stability low. It's not a spot where anyone expects topnotch scholarship. Yet Cole, as Bethel's special-ed director in the 1990s, initiated a program that has spurred a stunning rise in reading scores that has piqued the interest—and envy—of schools all over the country. What began as a casual remark in a taco joint emerged a year later as the Bethel Reading Project. Today, it's one of a select handful of federally designated K–3 model reading programs nationwide. In 2005, Bethel's Fairfield Elementary School was one of five Oregon schools and one district to be recognized by the state superintendent of public instruction for making significant progress toward closing the achievement gap between disadvantaged or minority students and their more affluent or nonminority peers.

At the small, struggling district, a team of academic researchers and a team of school practitioners set up a living laboratory. Reading experts at the University of Oregon joined forces with Bethel's teachers and administrators to implement, refine, and study a model of reading instruction that is gathering momentum in schools across the country: the "three-tier" model. The project goal is ambitious, especially for a bunch of kids from poor families—to make sure that every student, on the June afternoon when he waves his final good-bye to his third-grade teacher, is an able reader. This team of go-for-it educators plunged in with the same "just-do-it" spirit made famous by sports-and-fitness giant Nike, founded in this very town some forty years before.

Bethel's program reflects the growing chorus of experts, including the National Research Council, recommending the three-tier model, which is designed to prevent, diagnose, and treat reading problems. Among those recommending the approach is the National Association of School Psychologists, which argued for it in the latest reauthorization of IDEA this way:

Characteristic features of the multi-tiered model are as follows:
Tier 1: High-quality instructional and behavioral supports for all students in general education
Tier 2: Targeted intensive prevention or remediation services for students whose performance and rate of progress lag behind the norm for their grade and educational setting
Tier 3: Comprehensive evaluation by a multi-disciplinary team to determine eligibility for special education and related services

Three hundred miles to the north, University of Washington Professor Virginia Berninger and her multidisciplinary team of reading researchers are among the leading voices actively advocating for the model, which seeks to cut off most reading problems at the pass by attacking them early and aggressively. The idea is to blend science-based assessment and instruction in a continuous tapestry—assess and intervene, assess and modify, assess and treat. This tightly woven fabric of testing and teaching aims to keep nonreaders from slipping through school unnoticed, year after year. Under this plan, most kids will conquer reading in the regular classroom; only the most disabled readers will require diagnosis and special-ed placement.

The three-tier model is an efficient way to provide "differentiated instruction," which means, basically, meeting kids where they are. Instead of aiming instruction for some vague "middle" and hoping kids at the top and at the bottom will somehow benefit, the three-tier model allows teachers to tailor their teaching to give each child exactly what he needs to become a successful reader. The wide range of skills and experiences that children bring to school "requires a continuum of explicit instruction to create awareness of language processes," says Berninger. She and her colleagues argue that schools should redirect their attention from diagnosing "chronic failure" in reading and writing to intervening early with the goal of preventing failure before it happens. As described in the *Handbook of Psychoeducational Assessment* published by Academic Press (Berninger, Stage, Smith, and Hildebrand, 2001), the model works as follows:

Tier 1—Screening for early intervention: Every K–2 student in the school is screened to identify those who are at risk for reading and writing problems. The screening measures are brief, but research based. At-risk children get early intervention—but not just any intervention. It should be "science based," Berninger and her colleagues insist. By that they mean the real McCoy—a "theory-driven experiment in which competing hypotheses are tested" in search of "empirical evidence that an intervention is effective in improving student learning outcomes" (195).

Tier 2—Modifying the regular instructional program and monitoring the progress of students: The classroom program is modified for students who don't respond well to Tier 1 intervention. That modification might take a number of forms: adding curriculum components, changing teaching practices, revising materials, and/or providing extra skills practice. The goal of Tier 2 is to determine whether all the essential curriculum pieces are in place and being delivered effectively. To monitor progress, schools can use curriculum-based measurements. The process is guided by a multidisciplinary collaborative team using a problem-solving approach to make ongoing changes as needed. Because learning problems cut across disciplines and specialties, a team might include the school psychologist, the special educator, the speech and language pathologist, the social worker, the nurse, the principal, the Title I teacher, and the general-ed teacher.

Tier 3—Diagnosis and treatment of referred children: Students who failed to respond well to the first two tiers get a thorough assessment. The goals are to decide whether the child qualifies for special ed; to diagnose—based on current scientific knowledge—why the student is having trouble; and to design a systematic, coordinated treatment plan.

"Many reading and writing disabilities could be prevented or reduced in severity if a three-tier model of assessment for intervention were implemented in schools," Berninger and company assert. "The learning outcome for students with dyslexia and/or dysgraphia will be much better if schools do not wait until students fail for several years before beginning the process of assessment for intervention" (Berninger, Stage, Smith, and Hildebrand, 218).

To figure out which kids are at risk and need intervention in the Tier 1 phase, the researchers recommend short screenings like the two-minute tests developed by Marilyn Jager Adams, the Texas Primary Reading Inventory developed at the University of Texas-Houston Medical School, or DIBELS—Dynamic Indicators of Basic Early Literacy—developed at the UO. (For more examples, see the online "Reading Assessment Database for Grades K–2" compiled by the Southeast Educational Development Laboratory, www.sedl. org/reading/rad/database.html. Berninger, too, has developed an assessment instrument as part of the Process Assessment of the Learner package, the PAL Test Battery for Reading and Writing, which can be used at each tier of the model.)

At the Tier 3 stage, kids who haven't made gains despite the special help offered under Tier 1 or the curriculum tweaking done during Tier 2 should get an in-depth assessment for learning disabilities. Berninger recommends using what she calls a "multimodal" approach, one that draws on many sources, many tools—interviewing parents, for instance, as well as scouring student records, giving all sorts of tests (standardized, normed, and criterion-referenced), meeting with the student, and looking at portfolios and work samples.

UO researcher Kame'enui likes to describe the model as a "three-gated" system. Students who fail to respond to instruction at one level will move through the "gates" toward more intensive, more individualized instruction until they achieve success. Kame'enui stresses the necessity of alignment among the three tiers. "Three-tier programs," he says, "must be built on one single core program to avoid the mix-and-match problem of incompatible curriculums. As we say in Hawaii, the kid gets *kapakahi*—'mixed up'—when he's getting a little of this and a little of that." The Baltimore-based team of Robert E. Slavin and Nancy A. Madden, inventors of the reading curriculum Success for All (1989), use the more academic term "cognitive confusion" to describe the same phenomenon—baffling children by using multiple instructional approaches to reading, so that a child might get a phonics approach in the regular classroom, but a whole-language approach in a special-ed pullout (or vice versa).

As Joseph Torgesen writes in the *Journal of School Psychology*, prevention and early intervention are, very simply, essential for the well-being of kids. "The costs of waiting until mid-elementary school to identify children in need of special instruction in reading are simply too great," Torgesen said.

"There is the very sobering fact obtained in several longitudinal studies that children who are poor readers at the end of first grade almost never acquire average-level reading skills by the end of elementary school" (2002, 8).

It's Not Sorcery, It's Science

Rhonda Wolter could use a "time turner"—the magical device that gives Harry Potter's pal Hermione the power to solve her scheduling conflicts. In *The Prisoner of Azkaban,* book three of the J. K. Rowling series, Hermione startles her friends by popping up in one course on ancient runes and another on divination—simultaneously. If Wolter, like the studious Hogwarts witch, could be in two places at the same time, she wouldn't wear out so many heels or put in so many sixty-hour weeks.

What the reading coordinator for Oregon's Bethel School District lacks in potions and spells, however, she makes up with raw determination. Wolter's conviction—that every kid can learn to read if he gets the right kind of instruction—sustains her through all the skipped lunches and late nights.

Wolter started her career twenty-seven years ago teaching disadvantaged middle schoolers. As an "old-school" adherent to direct instruction, she had seen firsthand what struggling students could achieve with curriculums such as Corrective Reading and Reading Mastery, well taught. When she makes the rounds across this low-income district, she encounters hundreds of that rare species of American child: top readers whose families are in the bottom economic strata. She watches underprivileged first- and second-graders tear through hefty vocabulary words like "determination" and "suspended"— words that cause visitors to think they must have stumbled into a fourth-grade room by accident. She looks on as they dig into such classic folktales as "The Little Red Hen" and "The Boy Who Cried Wolf" with confidence and relish. Seeing those little readers wrestle successfully and happily with big words and big ideas gives her the elixir she needs to keep up her frenetic pace. But suggest that schools are impotent to overpower poverty and you'll sense the heat rising behind Wolter's usual sunniness.

"I picked up my NEA (National Education Association) magazine the other day and read a quote from a teacher who said, 'Well, of course our kids can't make progress because they're low income and they have tough homes,'" she says. "You know what? I can't buy that, and I don't buy it. And, you know why? Because our elementary schools have as many as 80 percent of the students on free or reduced-price lunch, yet they continue to produce awesome scores. Those kids are reading. So you can't tell me that kids can't do it for those reasons. It's not true. Come to Bethel and we'll show you."

Teachers and administrators from schools near and far are doing just that. Educational pilgrims flock to Bethel and perch in little chairs on the edges of classrooms, seeking to discover why 92 percent of Bethel third-graders, despite economic hardship and skimpy literacy experience from home, met state reading benchmarks in 2003–2004. One thing that strikes visitors instantly is the intensity of focus. Kids in K–3 classrooms are engaged, even riveted, as their teachers lead them through the complexities of print. The other thing that hits you is the rampant high-spiritedness. The little giggles that periodically ripple among the wiggly learners give the impression that reading and writing are up there with Barbie dolls and SpongeBob cartoons on the list of fun stuff to do. The buoyant atmosphere deflates the widely held idea that skills-based teaching bores kids to tears.

One morning late in the school year, veteran first-grade teacher Jan Johnson leads her nineteen students through a series of lively lessons. Part coach, part cheerleader, part stand-up comic, Johnson manages her class with equal measures of instruction, encouragement, and humor. Like so many gifted teachers, she possesses the energy of an NBA point guard, laced liberally with the patience of a scientist studying the life cycle of seventeen-year cicadas. Her affection for her little band of learners is evident both in her verbal language ("Good job, sweet pea!") and in her body language (a kindly touch on a tiny shoulder, a reassuring smile).

Blending her gifts as a teacher into her delivery of the research-based curriculum Open Court, Johnson succeeds, year after year, in bringing at-risk readers to grade level. Never mind that these little ones, with names like Siskiyou and Dakota, come from homes where Dad is an unemployed logger or Mom works two shifts at the diner to pay for space at the trailer court. Kids that might well have ended up in years of special ed, and eventually slipped away without a diploma to a life of illiteracy and poverty are, instead, waving their hands in the air to volunteer an answer. They *know* those answers. And it feels good.

"Who wants to spell elephant?" Johnson asks during a lesson on the *ph* sound. Together, the students come up with *elefant*.

"What needs to be fixed—one little thing?" the teacher prompts.

"The *f* needs to be a *ph*," Dylan asserts.

"Yes!" Johnson says, correcting the spelling on the board. "Our silly English language," she adds with an amused tsk-tsk. It's a refrain she sprinkles throughout the ninety-minute literacy block, a gentle and constant reminder to these novice readers that although the language follows logical rules a lot of the time, there are plenty of crazy exceptions and confusing spellings that just have to be learned. Johnson no longer accepts the whole-language notion that because English is not 100 percent phonetic—that is,

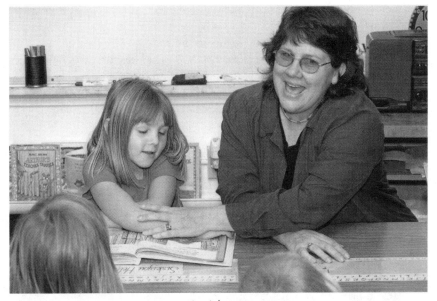

Jan Johnson

spellings aren't always predictable based on how words sound—kids (especially poor kids) will be confused and overwhelmed by the rules of spelling and grammar and by the deviations from those rules. That philosophy, she believes, doesn't give children enough credit. It seriously underestimates the capacity of the young child's intellect, the highly pliable brain that's capable of absorbing concepts of print like a two-ply paper towel.

"One big word for me is 'expectations,'" says Johnson, who trains other teachers in Open Court. "I did not believe, prior to this curriculum, that my kids could do this. But the curriculum gives us this magnificent framework. My kids have never been better writers, better readers."

Giggly Wigglers

Of course, Johnson cautions, you need to present those concepts in a child-friendly way—like when she gathers her first-graders, cross-legged on the frayed carpet at her feet, and holds up a white card with the words *hop on one foot* printed in black ink. Reminding them to read the messages silently to themselves, she tells them to follow the instructions printed on the card. First one student stands up and hops, and then a few more join in. Pretty soon, all the kids are up hopping. "What does it say?" Johnson prompts. "Hop on one foot!" the children chorus. Other cards appear in her hands: *hold nose, tap feet, wiggle fingers, laugh* ("Our silly English language!"). As Johnson calls their attention to the middle letters in the word *fingers* they chant, "i, n, g, i, n, g, ing, ing, ing!" in a catchy rhythm, their tiny torsos gyrating like rock stars'. The teacher extends the lessons to reinforce concepts already introduced. When the words *jump sideways* pop up, for example, the teacher asks, "Which one is a compound word?"

"Sideways!" is the response.

"What's a compound word?"

"A compound word is when two words are squished together to form one word," a student answers.

"Side!" Johnson calls out, raising one hand as the students follow her lead. "Ways!" Second hands go up. "Sideways!" they chorus, and then clap, once, in unison. The students volunteer other examples of compound words: *rainbow, into, outside, playground, birthday*. Then they come up with an array of words spelled with *ph*: *telephone, Joseph* (the name of one especially enthusiastic classmate), *photo*.

"Are we brilliant, or what?" Johnson rhapsodizes.

The Meaning of Things

The main missing piece in skills-based instruction, the critics charge, is meaning. Yet at Bethel, meaning is big. From start to finish during their 150-minute reading block, in both whole-group and small-group instruction, Johnson and her paraprofessional aides engage kids in discussions about the meanings of things. They delve into those meanings from the particular to the general, starting with definitions of individual words that turn up in daily reading selections. During a silly, rhyming story about a princess who wears a crown to bed, the word *royal* gets thoroughly discussed, as well as how a gown differs from a dress or a skirt. As usual, Johnson finds a way to inject humor and fun into the repartee, as in, "James, are you a prince?" James grins. His classmates titter delightedly. Another story prompts a dialogue about synonyms for sleep ("fancy words," as Johnson calls them), such as nap and snooze.

They also explore the meanings of stories as wholes. One selection, the classic folk tale "The Little Red Hen," illustrates the theme of someone who "keeps trying and trying and trying and never gives up," and includes clapping out syllables and identifying vowels for the word *determination*; the students are not the least bit daunted by the hefty word and its quintet of syllables. When Johnson asks the students, "What's a folk tale?" McKenzie's hand shoots up with rocket-like force. "It goes from generation to generation, family to family, friend to friend," the little girl responds smartly.

And, on an even more global level, the "theme of the week" serves as a conceptual wrapper that folds itself around all the literacy activities from Monday through Friday, giving unity to the week's vocabulary and readings. Working within the theme of "homes," for instance, one first-grade lesson not only introduces fresh lexicon but also explores world geography and anthropology. As Johnson's students browse a new reading selection, poring over the photos and descriptions of "Homes around the World" in their leveled Open Court Reading book, the tablemates buzz with the wonder over how people shelter themselves on the far reaches of the planet. A cliff house in Mali, a tin roof in Poland, stilts in the Philippines ("That's weird!" remarks Hope), a reed hut in Peru, a pueblo in New Mexico. The students even launch a spontaneous discussion about Australia versus Austria. The phonics—"sounding out" the novel words—is a tool the students use to find out things, like how some kids in rural Germany have grass growing on their roofs.

Is the phonics explicit? Yes. Is it systematic? Yes. Is it boring or stressful for Jesse and Joseph, Hope and Alicia? If it is, we never saw it. That isn't to say attention never wanders in these classrooms. Johnson gently brings daydreamers back to the task at hand. "You can't be sounding out if you're sleeping there, Bud," she tells one little fellow with a wandering gaze. "Show me your tracking finger."

A Pound of Prevention

An emphasis on phonics hasn't squelched this school's core concern: kids. In a cozy corner of Jan Johnson's room, racks and bins of books wrap around a kid-sized sofa and chair upholstered cheerily in ruby-red vinyl. A beagle named Ellie stretches and yawns on the frayed carpet, patiently submitting to hugs and pats as kids return from recess. For the privilege of walking the mellow beagle on the playground, students at Fairfield Elementary School work zealously to earn the required eight stickers. (Before Ellie, the school had a lovable pet pig named Petunia who liked to tuck her snout under students' arms and nuzzle.) A high school senior named Kyle, casually hip in his baseball cap and khaki shorts, is another favorite of Johnson's first-graders. Just being a teenager is enough to earn him the wide-eyed admiration of these little kids as he helps out in their classroom for his service-learning credit from Willamette High School.

A ChartPak at the front of the room displays word "families" for a week in late May:

Carry, carrot, narrow, barrel.
Parent, flare, glare, scare.
Berry, merry, terrible, cherry.

"Open Court gives you word families, which are just *phenomenal*," Johnson says. She loves Open Court—so much so, in fact, she has become a district trainer for other teachers.

Developed by Marilyn Jager Adams, author of the now classic work *Beginning to Read* published in 1990, Open Court is one of a growing number of reading materials that are based on current science and thoroughly tested for effectiveness. One district principal, Marilyn Martin, has a personal familiarity with Open Court that dates back twenty years, when she taught in Utah. After she used Open Court for two years in the mid-1980s, her district, as so many districts were doing at the time, dropped its skills-based approach in favor of whole language.

"I really felt like my students did much better with the phonics-based program," Martin reports.

When asked about the whole-language idea of creating readers by immersing kids in good books, this veteran educator says: "Well, I've never seen it work. You're not teaching them the skills to decode an unfamiliar word, to pull that word apart." But Martin concedes that phonics without literature is a little bit like vitamins without food: Vitamins may be vital to life, but it's the plate of steaming pasta primavera that makes the nutrients appetizing. In recognition of the need for real stories in the mix, skills-based programs like Open Court have moved toward a more global approach to reading—one that starts with, but goes beyond, what Martin calls the C-V-C (consonant, vowel, consonant) words that help kids learn but don't inspire them. "Open Court is doing a lot more with literature and comprehension now than it did back then," Martin says. "It has come along with the times, so that now we're teaching good literature along with the sounding out. From my perspective, literature is an important part of the mix because it gets kids excited about reading."

Open Court is one of the few products that have made the short list of materials approved by researchers Edward Kame'enui and Deborah Simmons of the University of Oregon, developers of a program they dubbed SRIM (Schoolwide Reading Improvement Model). Bethel joined forces with these researchers seven years ago in a sort of living laboratory. Kame'enui, then director of the university's Institute for Development of Educational Achievement, brought research to the school, and the teachers put the research into practice. Those teachers then gave their real-life findings back to the scholars. Together, the professors and the practitioners refined the model, posited other strategies, designed and piloted new studies, and analyzed results in a continuous feedback loop.

The model created by the UO researchers consists of five basic stages:

1. Big-picture (school-level) analysis
2. Individual (child-level) analysis
3. Instructional design
4. Goal setting and monitoring
5. Evaluation and modification

What truly drives the model is assessment—ongoing, regular, active assessment of students' reading skills. Three times a year, Bethel's staff of teachers and teacher assistants administers DIBELS (Dynamic Indicators of Early Basic Literacy), also of UO design. For kids who aren't yet meeting benchmarks, the assessment is more frequent. The developers christened the instrument "dynamic" because, unlike a standardized test that simply spits out a score, this assessment becomes the engine for placing a child precisely where she belongs and then moving her along in a fluid—dynamic— progression toward reading proficiency.

DIBELS, like other similar instruments designed to measure children's prereading and reading skills (such as the Texas Primary Reading Inventory and the PAL Test Battery for Reading and Writing), gives teachers a way to stay on top of their students' progress. It's really the ultimate in tailoring instruction to the individual needs of each and every kid because it gives teachers concrete, ongoing evidence of a child's strong points and weak areas.

"DIBELS gives you an awful lot of information in one minute," says the district's reading coordinator Rhonda Wolter. "We don't want to wait and find out *after* the statewide third-grade assessment that kids aren't getting it."

At the model's second stage, teachers perform "instructional triage." Borrowing the concept from emergency medical scenarios, in which nurses or EMTs prioritize treatment based on severity of need, the UO model builds in a three-tier system of grouping students based on their DIBELS scores— groupings that change frequently as regular assessments show lags or lurches in learning.

The model breaks down students' risk levels into three broad categories:

- Intensive—Students in acute need of intervention with "a sense of urgency" and twice-monthly monitoring with DIBELS
- Strategic—Students in need of systematic, strategic intervention and monthly monitoring
- Benchmark—Students on target, monitored thrice yearly

Fluid reading groups prevent ossification. Kids don't get embedded, like little handprints in clay that solidify and never change. Bethel's K–3 instructional groups cut across grade levels and span the entire range of reading readiness and skill development. Because its three-tier model meets kids on a full continuum of ability and disability, Bethel doesn't only *blur* the line between general and special education—nor does it, in fact, simply *erase* that line—but rather it actually *zaps* special education as a separate branch of schooling. Instead, special ed is folded in at one end of a continuum called, simply, "instruction."

Says Cole: "We have literally merged special ed and general ed."

Adds Wolter: "We all work together. It's not 'your kids' versus 'my kids'—they're *our* kids."

Marilyn Martin, principal of Fairfield Elementary School, explains it this way: "Unless it's a glaring problem, we really stay away from identifying any of our kindergarten or first-grade students for special ed. This year, in fact, we've identified zero special-ed students in those grades."

That is not to say that kids in the Bethel School District never get identified as learning disabled or that they never receive special-ed services. They do. But the proportion of second-graders getting an IEP has shrunk by two-thirds since the start of the program—from about 15 percent to around 5 percent.

"The district has historically had a very high number of kids who were identified for special ed," says Cole. "One day, the superintendent asked me, 'Why do you have so many kids in special ed? Why is special ed growing?' I gave him a flippant comeback: 'We don't recruit, you know! We don't call the principals up and say, Gee, our numbers are down. Can you send some kids to us?' "

Bethel's incredible shrinking special-ed population includes all kinds of physical, emotional, and developmental disabilities, as well as those who have a biologically based learning disability, usually dyslexia. But now there's a whole new category of kids—kids who once-upon-a-time *would* have ended up with a special-ed label but now get intensive, early intervention to prevent reading failure before it happens. These are kids who have been stymied, not by a brain glitch but by an instructional glitch.

"So many kids who are in special education are there because they didn't have the opportunity to learn," says Cole. "Deb Simmons calls them 'instructional casualties.' In my early career as a special-ed teacher in middle school, the majority of LD kids were sitting in the back of the classroom with their jackets on and their hats on, because school was not a good place for them."

Instead of facing a future of slouching in the back row, struggling readers at Bethel are getting a "double dose" or even a triple dose of reading instruction, usually before or after school, starting as soon as assessments reveal deficits. Johnson, who treats kids from her intensive group to a "fun little book club" two afternoons a week, is passionate about the importance of first-grade reading development. "They are in trouble if they don't have skills," she says. "We do everything we can to give them that little oomph."

Principal Jane Carter of Bethel's Meadow View Elementary School concurs. "If we didn't do that, they would be LD, I guarantee it. They would be LD for life."

Bethel is doing what most educators agree is right, but few schools actually pull off: prevention. By tackling troubles hard and fast from day one of kindergarten, most kids at risk of reading problems miss out on those problems completely, never becoming what Simmons calls "instructional casualties."

Drew Braun, Bethel's main data cruncher, jokes grimly that if educators were subject to the same kinds of legal liability as medical doctors, the victims of poor instruction would be "the malpractice lawsuits." That's because the typical U.S. school has adopted the "wait-to-fail" mode, which forces kids to undergo the scarring anguish, the emotional ravaging, that reading failure inflicts. By the time the school recognizes that the fissure between IQ and achievement has become a gaping crevasse—typically in third grade, but often as late as middle school—the struggling reader is all too likely to be depressed and dejected, angry and antagonistic, fearful and frustrated.

Behavioral problems piggyback upon the academic distress. Historically, the IQ-achievement discrepancy has been the ticket to services for struggling kids, as mandated by federal special-education law. At this writing, lawmakers have recently hammered out a revision of that law, to be implemented in the schools beginning in the fall of 2005. Meanwhile, districts such as Bethel have found in the three-tier model a way to save countless kids from ever knowing reading failure, let alone seeing the inside of a special-ed resource room.

Benchmark Bonanza

The scenes a visitor might see as she tours the district's six Open Court schools include:

- After reading "The Little Red Hen" in the Open Court anthology ("I *love* this one!" Kirstin remarks), Jan Johnson's first-graders engage in a verbal ramble about all aspects of the classic story—the laziness of the hen's canine, feline, and rodent compatriots, the dog, the cat, and the mouse. About the meaning of the word "cozy." About grinding wheat in a mill to make bread. "How do you turn wheat into a flower?" Johnson asks playfully. "Not *that* kind of flower!" a student snorts in a tone of exasperation. Explains another child, "It's the flour that's white and soft and comes in a bag!"

- In an after-school "double dose" class, groups of three or four kinder-gartners are working on the letter *z*, little tongues against baby teeth: "Zzzzzzzz—zebra!" Each child gets a card stamped with a *z* and a series of pictures. After tracing the letter with their fingers, the students pick out the images that start with *z*—zoo, zipper, zebra. "OK, everyone say zzzzzzzz—zebra!" the teacher assistant says. "Excellent! Way to go!"

- In an Open Court "booster" session, a teacher assistant prompts an interpretation of "The Boy Who Cried Wolf" with a series of questions about character, plot, and message. "Why didn't the villagers come?" she queries. Miranda replies promptly. "Because the boy kept tricking them, so they thought he was tricking them again," she volunteers. Asks the teacher: "What lesson did the boy learn?" Answers Miranda, "Not to trick the villagers!"

Shouting Out Loud

Back when the district adopted its new science-based reading materials, K–8 Meadow View was the maverick. There, teachers chose Reading Mastery instead of Open Court. Although the program, published by SRA/McGraw-Hill, is more cut-and-dried than Open Court, the students at Meadow View look as happy and engaged as those at the Open Court schools. The teachers appear equally encouraging, nurturing, and fun loving. The level of learning is as high as the spirits.

Look in on one room, a second- and third-grade mix. Crackling with energy on an overcast day in May, the class is engaged in a discussion of the word "suspended," which appears in a story they have been studying. Together, the students and teacher suggest multiple meanings: something hanging in the air, something an old farmer would wear to hold up his pants, something that could happen to a student who messes up in school.

"Absolutely! Like, totally, man," the young teacher enthuses, tongue in cheek.

Then she picks up a bongo drum and, in a rhythm that is at once soothing and invigorating, she taps out a cadence to encourage fluency as the students read in chorus. When the readers stumble on the word "lighting," she talks them through it, calling their attention to the spelling and the meaning, con-trasting it to the word "lightning." As the class warms to the reading, the teacher drums faster, pushing their fluency rates to greater speeds. The young readers keep right up.

Next they turn to a story titled "Winter at the North Pole." Just about every student in the room has a hand aloft, volunteering to read a passage aloud. As her classmates track the text with their fingers, Janelle reads with brisk confidence, "The air was so bitter he could hardly breathe . . " Another student, reading from a passage containing dialogue, inflects the words of one character with a convincing Indian accent to suggest the character's Near East ancestry. When a third girl trips over a sentence, the teacher intercedes with a correction, and the student rereads the section. A scientific discussion then ensues about what causes winter. In the midst of a classwide exchange about the earth's jaunty tilt and its yearly spin around the sun, Kara raises her hand, and, interjecting a glaring non sequitur, asks, "Can I bring my African drum to school so you can drum every day?" The teacher smiles indulgently and says, "Sure, Kara," before moving along to choral spelling of key words from the text they just read. Kids with names like Shania and Savannah, Devon and Jalan belt out the spellings with a clear intent to out-yell the kid sitting beside them. The students' obvious joy at getting to shout in school—and vent some pre-recess energy—gives this spelling lesson the feel of a pep rally, once again giving the lie to the idea that skills instruction saps schooling of fun.

Meadow View's scores confirm the program's success: 91 percent of the school's third-graders met or exceeded state reading standards in 2003.

The bongo as a fluency-building tool—a huge hit with kids—shows how a teacher's creativity can converge with a structured, science-based curriculum such as Reading Mastery. Off-the-shelf reading programs have met with fierce attack from many teachers who see them as a threat to their individuality, spontaneity, and professionalism. Principal Marilyn Martin argues that a systematic, science-based program's greatest strength—its airtight coverage of beginning reading skills—is in no way incompatible with inspired teaching. "Open Court doesn't leave holes, it doesn't leave gaps," she says. "But you can follow the program and be creative at the same time."

As an example, she tells about one second-grade teacher in her building who "gets her freedom of expression" by layering extra subject-area material on top of the Open Court literature selections, smoothly segueing from those stories into science and social science lessons. Thus, the Open Court story forms the spool from which unwinds a thematic thread for an entire day's instruction. One interdisciplinary unit she designed, for instance, unfolded from a story on fossils. Jan Johnson, during a read-aloud one day, picked up on her students' fascination with turtles. So for the next two months, she steeped her teaching in turtle lore, turtle literature, turtle science—"love of turtle," is the way she puts it.

Johnson argues that it's unrealistic to expect each teacher to design his or her own reading program from scratch, particularly when most teacher candidates get very little training in how to teach reading. "Our district says, 'Don't reinvent the wheel,'" she explains. "Open Court gives us this marvelous framework. The pacing, the timing, the transitions are absolutely phenomenal. But it's *not* a script."

As Johnson guides kids through the minefield of English literacy, deftly disarming such hazards as silent letters and irregular spellings, she looks and sounds like anything but a preprogrammed robot. Yes, the instruction is explicit, direct, and skills based. But it's also challenging, cerebral, and highly interactive. Not even the trickiest alphabetic booby trap causes Johnson to veer from the task of making readers.

On this particular day, she ventures into the scary linguistic territory of words ending in *-tion*. Unintimidated by the illogical pronunciation (*-shun*), she forges ahead and the students gamely follow. Next, they move on to a review of words starting with a silent *w*—*wrist, wreck, wreath,* and *wriggle*—and then contrast these with regular *r* words like *ring* and *ragged*. They segment words and blend them together. Holding up one finger for each letter sound, they review which two letters make a /k/ sound at a word's end (-ck) and then spell truck, tick, and trick. They go over the /sh/ sound at the end of a word, and then spell hash, cash, and fish. They do quick reviews of *-ing* (as in fishing) and *-th* (as in with), once again holding up a finger for each letter sound. After the lively session in which kids are actively engaged in working out spellings, clapping out syllables, inventing sentences, reading aloud in chorus and individually, discussing word meanings, and pondering story themes, Johnson ends the lesson with one of her verbal megavitamins: "You guys are brilliant today! Whew!"

One of the key predictors for reading success, researchers at UO have found, is fluency—that is, how quickly and smoothly the child can read. As Johnson notes, "To be good a comprehender, you have to read with automaticity." That's because if you have to labor over every word, you've forgotten the first one by the time you get to the end of the sentence. Meaning gets lost in the tedium of code breaking.

To measure kids' ability to read with fluidity, teachers at Bethel count words per minute as students read aloud as part of the ongoing DIBELS assessments. Johnson has seen her first-graders' fluency rates rocket skyward as her own skill with Open Court has developed. At the end of the baseline year—the initial year of testing with DIBELS, pre–Open Court—found her kids reading thirty-four words per minute. The next year, after Open Court was launched, her kids' reading rate had climbed to fifty-eight words per minute. In 2003, after four years with the program, Johnson's end-of-year first-graders were averaging almost ninety-three words per minute—nearly three times the fluency rate she had achieved in the old days. The UO researchers have found that kids who read 114 words a minute at the end of third grade have a 97.5 percent chance of meeting state benchmarks in reading. It looks like Jan Johnson's first-graders are on their way not only to meeting but bursting beyond those goals.

As the students work on a writing project at their tables, Johnson looks across the classroom and indicates a golden-skinned girl whose desk placard reads Sheecid. "That little girl started here in October," she tells us. "She came from Mexico with zero English. Now she reads 101 words a minute."

For Johnson, Sheecid's achievement is a staggering piece of hard evidence. "I'm putting *my* faith," she says, "in research."

Johnson's faith in science is, however, outside the American educational mainstream. Acknowledging teachers' widespread resistance to the body of knowledge about reading accumulating in fields such as psychology, neurology, and pediatrics, as well as education, Carl Cole shakes his head in exasperation.

"It just amazes me," he says, and then lets a note of sarcasm creep into his voice. "We're educators, but we're not supposed to use the knowledge base? We have incredible research—thirty years of research—in reading. Right here in Bethel, we can show you five years of research showing a dramatic decrease in the number of kids who are identified for special education. We can show you a steady increase in the number of kids who are at benchmark. We can show you that if kids are on target on the DIBELS at the end of kindergarten, they have a 97 percent chance of meeting the benchmark when they reach third grade. It's science. Does it *feel* good? I don't know. The other day, one teacher told me that when she came to Meadow View, which is our Reading Mastery school, she was a whole-language teacher. And she was *positive* that that is how kids learn. So she collected the data for the year for one reason and one reason only: to prove her principal wrong. She said, 'At the end of the year, I'm like, "Oh, my goodness!" ' "

"I don't need to make a religion out of it, but in education, there are only a few things we know, that we really can say with confidence. We know grade-school reading. It's not negotiable anymore. We know how kids read. We know that if you have them on track by the end of third grade, they're going to keep going."

"PEOPLE HAVE MISUNDERSTOOD
HOW READING DEVELOPS"

Even on the grayest Oregon day, the high-ceilinged foyer at Meadow View Elementary School is flooded with daylight, captured by big windows that

Table 5.1. Fairfield Student Performance
(Percent meeting and exceeding benchmarks)

Grade	Reading & Literature 1998–99	Reading & Literature 2003–04
3	72%	93%
5	54%	83%

Table 5.2. Fairfield 2003–04 Student Performance by Subpopulations
(Percent meeting and exceeding benchmarks)

	Grade 3 Reading & Literature	
Subpopulations	Fairfield	State Average
Hispanic	85%	63%
Econ. Disadvantaged	91%	73%
Special Education	87%	52%

	Grade 5 Reading & Literature	
	Fairfield	State Average
Hispanic	69%	54%
Econ. Disadvantaged	80%	65%
Special Education	69%	42%

Table 5.3. Relationship between Oral Reading Fluency and Performance on the
Oregon Reading & Literature Assessment
(Percent of students who meet the benchmark)

Instructional Category	Intensive	Low Reader	Emerging Reader	Established Reader
Grade 3 ORF	0–40 wpm	40–69 wpm	70–119 wpm	120+ wpm
Grade 3 Meets/Exceeds	0%	29.1%	81.4%	97.6%
Grade 5 ORF	0–60 wpm	60–99 wpm	100–149 wpm	150+
Grade 5 Meets/Exceeds	0%	56.5%	87.2%	98.8%

frame the fields surrounding this innovative K–8 school. The woman who leads Meadow View emits her own radiance as she strides out of her office to shake our hands with a powerful grip that is both warm and businesslike. That potent combination—a serious commitment to the business of learning, wrapped in a nurturing blanket of care for kids—defines Jane Carter's vision as principal.

Consider, for example, the bright yellow "CAT CROSSING" sign posted

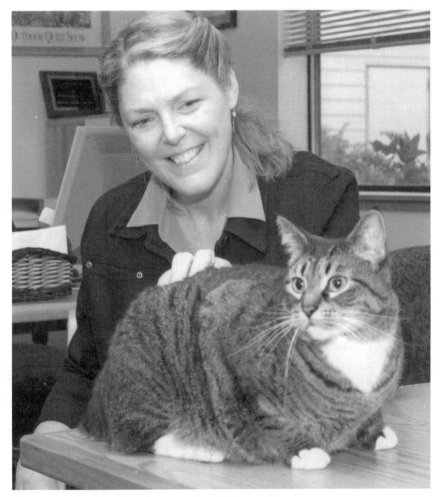

Jane Carter

outside Carter's office. The sign is a tongue-in-cheek warning for pedestrians to keep an eye out for Jackson, a supersized tabby who strolls in and out between naps. The green-eyed mascot gives the administrative offices, quite literally, a warm, fuzzy feeling. But a conversation with Carter quickly dispels any idea that a critter, no matter how chubby and cuddly, could distract her from her dead-serious mission: ensuring the academic success of the 850 mostly disadvantaged students in her charge.

With a PhD in special education from the University of Oregon, Carter is a longtime adherent of the direct-instruction model, especially for kids at risk of failure. She knows this approach draws a lot of flak from educators who've been trained in the whole-language and developmental models. Leaning over to give Jackson an affection pat, she jokes, "We're *not* the Gestapo."

Q: What reading materials and approaches were your teachers using before the school switched to Reading Mastery?

CARTER: It was pretty much a hodge-podge of materials, especially in the kindergarten program. There was nothing systematic about it. It was the letter-of-the-week kind of approach to reading and lots of games and songs about letters and sounds, coloring pages, word walls—very eclectic. There were lots of Big Books and read-alouds and stories—kind of what I would think of today as the preschool approach. Then, in first and second grades, we used a literature-based or whole-language basal, so again more stories and read-alouds, Big Books. There were some words in isolation, very little in the way of phonics, except for some individual teachers who preferred that style.

Q: So some teachers taught phonics?

CARTER: Yes, but not systematically. And there was no measurement system at all—no feedback to the teachers about specific skills and whether their kids were getting it until the state assessments at the end of third grade. Then there was a big surprise.

Q: Philosophically, early childhood educators have tended to oppose any sort of academic approach with kindergartners.

CARTER: Very much. It was just not in our lexicon to think that five-year-olds could read. It was not in our understanding about how five-year-olds' brains work. Many folks resisted the idea. They said, "It's too much, it's too hard, they're not ready. Gosh, kids are supposed to play in kindergarten and primary school and have fun and take a nap if they're tired." The catch-phrase that is used a lot is "developmentally appropriate practices." Reading Mastery is a very systematic, say-it-together kind of approach to reading. Many people react by saying: "Oh, no, this will just ruin reading for children. They'll hate it." I've heard that a lot. People needed to be convinced. I hate to use the catch-phrase "paradigm shift," but that really is what happened here.

Q: There's a lot of resistance, as well, about methods that use direct instruction, and in particular the "signaling" used by teachers in Reading Mastery.

CARTER: When people observe a class and see the teacher snapping her fingers or the children saying things out loud together, they can perceive it as some kind of mechanical experience. I think it's a huge misconception. You and I, as adult readers, approach literature differently than an emerging reader does. We have a lot to bring to the books we read and a different level of understanding of literature. My favorite thing to do is read, but that's because I'm a good reader. I think people have misunderstood how reading develops. The National Reading Panel's work is beginning to change our understanding of what kids need to be good readers. It's not just having rich literature. I wish that were true. My sense is that there is quite a bias around having kids sound out words and controlled vocabulary at the very earliest parts of Reading Mastery because the controlled vocabulary results in sort of artificial stories. At the very youngest and earliest stages of Reading Mastery, the stories are kind of dry because they are controlled. They sound contrived. It's not the rich literature that we love and that we think children would love. But I'm telling you that the kids love to read because they *can* read. They feel competent. They're not bored by the stories. The stories are corny, but the kids are having fun with it. The belief that kids won't love reading if they go through direct instruction is truly a misconception.

Q: How did you go about convincing teachers?

CARTER: The beauty of what happened is that I didn't have to convince them. One of the first-grade teachers we hired had been teaching direct instruction for many years and asked if she could use it. I said it was fine. That year we started using DIBELS assessment. By the second year, that teacher's DIBELS scores far exceeded the others'. That's all it took. Teachers looked at the evidence of learning, and they were convinced—or at least intrigued enough to say: "What did she do? How come she got such good results?" By the third year, the teachers became convinced that Reading Mastery might be the approach they wanted. I secured a couple of Goals 2000 grants for training all the kindergarten, first-grade, and second-grade teachers. Staff development is critical to the implementation of Reading Mastery. It's a very technical program. Over the next two years, we very systematically worked with the National Institute for Direct Instruction. We hired an implementation consultant, who works with us today. I don't really have to convince anyone of its effectiveness. They just look at the data. Each time we do our DIBELS data collection three times a year, they just can't wait to see it. There is excitement about successes they'd never seen before. Each year, our kids' performance gets better and better. In the ninety minutes we teach reading, we have fourteen different levels of Reading Mastery going on simultaneously. Kids develop at different rates no matter what their age is, but because we have these levels of instruction available, they can work at their own rate and advance as fast as they can.

Q: One criticism of direct instruction and explicit phonics is that kids who are great readers don't need all that instruction in skills. How do you answer those critics?

CARTER: We were very sensitive to that criticism early on. Because we're carefully collecting the data—three times a year with DIBELS and the mastery tests built into the program—we monitor that. We accelerate kids just as quickly as we can. There is no reason for kids to go over known territory, to get bored with it. But the difference is that it's a data-based decision. You can look at a kid who has passed all her mastery tests for the last five checkouts, her reading rates are faster than we expected, and then we can look across these fifteen or sixteen instructional groupings and see where the match is. We have third-graders in Level 6, which is fifth-grade material. We have a kindergartener in third-grade material. Unfortunately, we also have second-graders in kindergarten material because they're not making the progress. Kids sitting next to each other might include one kid who is LD-identified, another kid who is a nonidentified youngster, and a Title I kid. Reading is becoming a continuum—it's not third-grade reading, second-grade reading, or first-grade reading. That's a barrier. If you run Reading Mastery in a grade-orientated deployment, you're going to have those problems. I think in any program, you have to break out of that grade assignment. We put kids where their ability is, not their grade assignment.

Q: So the LD kids are part of the regular group instruction, right? They're simply placed in a group that matches their skill level.

CARTER: Yes. It's the inclusion model for reading in K–3. No one would know who the special-ed teachers are or who the special-ed kids are. You don't need to worry about that. The IEP goals are met. We have a student who has moved up about three or four instructional groups since October, a second-grader who didn't have a background in Reading Mastery, but who has moved up because he's got it now. We don't keep him going on sound-outs because we don't need to. We see he's got it and his fluency rates have developed all year long. It's fun and a very dynamic thing to watch

Q: What happens after third grade?

CARTER: By fourth grade, we go back to more of a literature-based approach, and in middle school, an integrated language arts/social studies block approach. So teachers are free to use pretty sophisticated novels and literature that integrates with their social studies. Because the district is five or six years into this reading program, you can look at the data and basically draw a line between when we started Reading Mastery and Open Court. For the kids who are starting middle school now, their ability to do the reading is fundamentally better than the eighth-graders who didn't have the explicit phonics. The thing that is so crazy making is that you *know* what happened to kids who struggle in middle school. You *know* that this kid never got the code, never got it unlocked, and has struggled every year. It's sad to watch.

6

It's Never Too Late: Rescuing Struggling Readers at Any Age

How do we help kids at older ages with all the baggage they're carrying begin to get over the hump?

> —Reid Lyon, National Institutes of Health
> "Children of the Code," 2004

Adults invariably harbor deep pain and sadness reflecting years of assaults to their sense of self-worth.

> —Sally Shaywitz
> *Overcoming Dyslexia*

The adolescents show us a level of pain that this society doesn't even see.

> —Reid Lyon, National Institutes of Health
> "Children of the Code," 2004

Dan Anderson's story could be the story of a million children. Like every true story, the details of time and place and name are unique. Yet to kids and families devastated by reading disability, the sequence of events will seem as familiar as a favorite bedtime story.

THE STORY OF DAN, AS TOLD BY LEE SHERMAN

We look in on Dan's life as it was in the mid-1990s. He was a fifth-grader, a good-looking, revved-up, funny kid who could mimic Arnold Schwarzeneg-

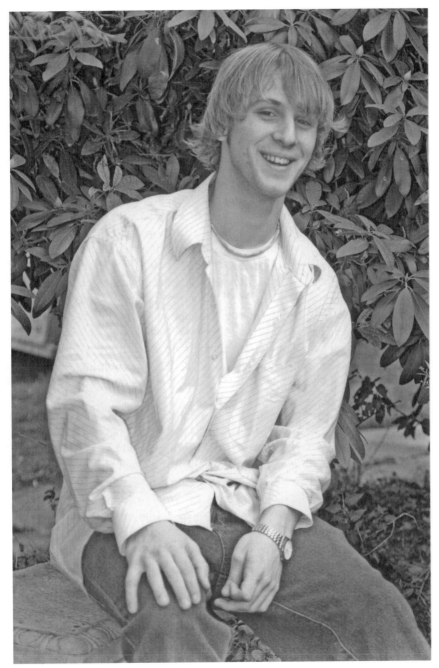

Dan Anderson

ger's "Hasta la vista, baby!" with just the right swagger and Homer Simpson's "Doe!" with perfect cluelessness. A committed videophile, he had a steel-trap memory for movie dialog and would annoy other viewers by blurting out the lines to *Toy Story* and *The Adventures of Huck Finn* in advance of the actors. He could tell you excruciatingly fine details about the hot cars and the bling-bling of every rap star. The history and mystery of medieval Europe tugged at his curiosity. He'd check out stacks of picture books on castles and ancient warfare, studying the drawings of ramparts and chain mail, moats and truncheons, until the library called with an overdue notice.

His dad and I, tired of dating, had bought a big old house where we could all live together as a family. I knew Dan had a reading problem, but it was only after becoming his de facto stepmom that I began to understand how stuck he really was. Opening a book without pictures gave him the sensation of stepping into the deep black muck of a reedy bog: You feel the ooze close around your foot like wet cement. As you try to pull free, the mud tightens with a sickening sucking sound. So mired, Dan was in a constant state of panic. He picked fights with his younger brother (an excellent reader), threw a lot of tantrums, and screamed bloody murder over injuries as small as a sliver or a stubbed toe. He was scared. And he was hurting.

I started to feel guilty making him go off to school every morning. He would dawdle and complain about an aching head or an upset stomach. He looked so miserable as he slouched off to the bus stop wearing a backpack bulging with books he couldn't read. I had a lump in my throat as I called out hopefully, "Have a good day!"

Then came the turning point—that autumn day when Dan blew up. As I think back on it now, Dan's experience at his new school bears an uncomfortable likeness to those scenes from *The Wild Kingdom* where a pride of lions, crouching, circling, then crashing through the savannah, takes down a wounded wildebeest. His classmates, having seen his halting efforts to read, had pounced. They shunned him on the playground, so he sat on the sidelines. At lunch, the other boys pushed him and mocked him, refusing to let him sit down. He had to eat with the girls. On this particular day, as a crush of students pushed through the halls after recess, a boy from our new neighborhood—Dan's only friend at his new school—joined the chorus of voices hissing "dummy!" in Dan's direction. His rage and shame spewed out in a spasm of flying fists. He punched his friend.

When the principal asked Dan to write down his version of events, his explanation looked something like this: "*gdncldmedmndihthmm.*" His friend, who at that moment seemed to us like the worst kind of Benedict Arnold, had in fact done Dan a favor. The crux of the problem was right there in black and white.

At home that night, Dan sat on his dad's lap and cried bitterly, sobbing as though his heart was broken. "I *hate* my life, I *hate* my life," he moaned, tears streaking his pale cheeks. "Dad, get a gun and shoot me. Just shoot me."

Today, more than eight years later, that scene—a sturdy, ten-year-old boy folded limply in his daddy's arms, wailing in despair—is clearer in my mind than this morning's bowl of oatmeal. We know now that Dan was struggling with a problem much deeper than simply lagging behind. But in the beginning, Daniel's dad (then a single parent trying to hold things together alone) accepted the first- and second-grade teachers' assurances that Dan would "catch up." When Dan wasn't reading by third grade, the school assigned him to the resource room for a half-hour of remediation each day. Pretty soon, Dad was running Dan to private remedial classes, evenings and summers, and footing the bill. The lead teacher at this alternative school saw in Dan classic signs of dyslexia, especially his inability to link letters with sounds—to make the connection between print and speech. But when Dan's dad requested that the school district test him for a learning disability, he was told that Dan was already getting all the extra help that was available, so an LD ID would be moot.

When I started dating Dan's dad, I'd drive up to their house on school nights and spot the two of them through the kitchen window, heads together at the old Formica table, Dan's forehead scrunched in concentration over a schoolbook.

"I couldn't remember anything they tried to teach me," Dan recalls of those early years. "After a while, I just didn't pay attention. I would always say I was sick, that I had a tummy ache or something."

After Dan's blowup at school and emotional meltdown at home, we pulled him from school until the district could come up with a better plan than sink-or-swim. A battery of tests revealed a huge discrepancy between his IQ (normal) and his achievement level (somewhere between first and second grade). Dan had a learning disability.

This is where Dan's story is likely to diverge from that of the typical LD child. That's because, serendipitously, Portland Public School District had just that year launched a program tailor-made for kids like Dan—bright children whose brain wiring makes learning to read exceedingly difficult. Dan was placed in the district's new ILC—Intensive Learning Center—a class of twelve LD kids with a teacher skilled in direct instruction and an instructional assistant to ensure that kids got lots of individual help. As I drove Dan across town to his first day at his new school, he looked out the window while our minivan cruised across the Marquam Bridge, downtown Portland glowing in the morning sun. "I'm going to go to Harvard," he announced. "Great!" I said. "And Stanford," he added. I smiled. A few minutes later he said, "I'm going to be a doctor. And a lawyer." This was the kid who only a few weeks before had complained, scowling, about facing a certain future as a garbage collector.

Dan stayed in the ILC through seventh grade. "I remember *aaa, aye, awe*—we had to sound out every letter, like, a million times," Dan, who's now eighteen, says as he recalls his years in the ILC. "I remember learning the rules and stuff—the magic *e* rule, like in "came": you don't hear the *e*, but it makes the *a* say its name. I remember learning sight words—little words like 'it.'"

I asked him if it was boring, having to focus on all those little tiny pieces of written English. "Half the time it was," he said after thinking about it for a minute. "But you could tell you were learning stuff because you could remember it. You had to learn the whole alphabet and all the rules first, but by the middle of the year it all started to make sense. I was the fastest reader in the class, and I was the best reader in the class, and I got all this confidence. And I started getting better and better."

To supplement the instruction he was getting in school, we hired a tutor who was trained to work with dyslexic kids. Using Orton-Gillingham multi-sensory instruction, along with her big library of juvenile literary works, she accelerated Dan's reading gains.

Even though Dan was finally making progress in academics, the emotional toll from his earlier failures constantly thwarted his progress in life, both in and out of school. He became ultra-fastidious about his appearance. We knew it had gone beyond the normal adolescent obsession with hair and clothes when we noticed him getting up extra early on school days to iron his shirts, jeans—even his undershirts. One morning when I stopped by his room to check on his progress, I saw him carefully pressing his white socks. Feigning nonchalance until I left his room, I hurried downstairs and found his dad reading the paper. I whispered, "Daniel is ironing his *socks!*" We conferred anxiously over this new development. What kind of weird compulsion, we wondered, would cause a teenage boy to iron his crew socks, especially in the age of "grunge"? But a few days later when I mentioned this worrisome behavior to Dan's tutor, she instantly put it in perspective. "Oh, of course," she said. "He's making sure no one can ever find fault with him again—no wrinkles, no stains. He needs to feel a sense of perfection when he presents himself to the world. No one will ever mock him again—not if *he* can help it."

Like a lot of kids who aren't making it academically, Dan tried on all sorts of hats to win acceptance from his peers—class clown, rebel, cut-up, loud-mouth, smart-ass, hotshot, stoner. He got kicked out of high school, and we enrolled him in a small, enlightened community school where classes are small, teachers are demanding but nurturing, and students range from brilliant, artistic, and gifted to geeky, gawky, disgruntled, and, like Dan, learning disabled. Dan is thriving there, where kindness is the one absolute. For a recent writing assignment to describe "the most peaceful place you've ever been," Dan's essay on snowboarding began like this:

> Literally chillin' in a cushy La-Z-Boy made of powdery snow. It seems I was just smashing down the mountain like an avalanche. I turn toe-side on a bend in the run and catch a glimpse. An uncontrollable force tosses me into the pillowy snow chair with ease, and I sit flabbergasted by the sight in front of me. On the highest point of Mt. Hood I have ever been, the world is revealed to me. Pure beauty is the only way to describe it. As the sun rises higher in the sky, an astonishing and unfathomable blast of color, shadow, and nature pierces my sight. I am dumbfounded by not only the sight but the feeling—the feeling of me on a mountain ready for a wonderful day of snowboarding, hanging out with friends, and growing closer. While I sit in comfort, I try to guess how many miles of life lay before me. I think 50, 70, 100. I don't know.

His senior year, Dan traveled with an Israeli friend to the Middle East, where he spent Christmas break in the Mediterranean city of Haifa. At this writing, he is working on his senior dissertation—a multimedia presentation on Israeli youth culture. And he reads. When we can't find him, chances are he's hunkered down in the bathtub, immersed in hot water and a good book.

These days, when I drop Dan off at Pacific Crest Community School, it's he who calls out cheerfully, "Have a good day!" His chin is up, his shoulders are straight. He can read the books bulging in his backpack—even if he doesn't always read them on deadline.

SOMNOLENT SAMANTHA

As Dan's story shows, "It is never too late to remediate," in the words of University of Washington researchers Sylvia Abbott and Virginia Berninger. In a 1999 study by that name, Abbott and Berninger found that "upper elementary and middle school students responded positively to instructional interventions that emphasized linguistic awareness and executive functions."

But such findings will not help kids as long as educators cling to the old myths and misconceptions about reading disabilities. One of these misconceptions—and one which kids quickly internalize—is that reading ability is a proxy for intelligence. While researching this book, we ran into people over and over who said something like this: "Oh, yeah, I have a nephew [or a cousin or a friend] who is dyslexic. It's so odd, because his brother is so bright." And virtually every dyslexic person we interviewed said, "My big sister [or my little brother] was smart—she could read." The subtext: "Kids who learn to read easily have more natural brain power than kids who wrestle with written words." Research, however, is unequivocal: Reading disability is in no way tethered to how smart you are. Kids with IQs both low and high can have dyslexia or struggle with print, including those we would judge to be geniuses.

Another pernicious and tenacious myth that chips away at kids' self-concept is that there's really no such thing as brain-based learning disabilities. When Dan's stepmom was conferring with his sophomore English teacher about his problems finishing writing assignments in class, she said, "Well, Dan's dyslexic, you know." The teacher just stared at her for a moment, and then said, dismissively, "He's just bored." Despite the growing body of compelling research that, quite literally, captures photographic images of brain differences in LD kids, doubters abound. In a chapter for the *Handbook of Child Psychology* (2006), Berninger writes, "I am not being facetious when I characterize my line of research as studying a phenomenon that schools do not believe exists."

The most notorious example of this denial of dyslexia in recent years centered around the president of a top university who not only refused certain accommodations to LD students but also mounted a mean-spirited vendetta against them. The ridicule and mockery this academician heaped on disabled students landed him in court, as well as on a segment of *Good Morning, America* and in the pages of the *New York Times*.

Jon Westling was president of Boston University in 1995 when he decided, arbitrarily, to cut some of the accommodations that the university's renowned Learning Disabilities Support Services had been providing for years. Then, in a series of speeches, he lambasted what he called the "learning disabilities movement." To illustrate his points, he described a student named Somnolent Samantha who, he said, had a habit of dozing off in class and then asking the professor to fill her in on what she had missed, along with demanding a note-taker and a laundry list of other accommodations. It turned out, however, that Somnolent Samantha was a figment of Westling's prejudices. He admitted during the trial of *Elizabeth Guckenberger et al.* vs. *Boston University et al.*, a class-action suit brought by LD students in 1997, that not only had he invented her, she wasn't even *patterned* after a real student at BU or anywhere else.

In its Findings of Fact, Conclusions of Law, and Order of Judgment dated August 15, 1997, the court painted a disturbing portrait of a college administration that was dangerously ill-informed about learning disabilities and, worse, steeped in damaging stereotypes. Wrote U.S. District Court Judge Patti B. Saris, "'Somnolent Samantha' represented Westling's belief—fueled mostly by popular press and anecdotal accounts—that students with learning disabilities were often fakers who undercut academic rigor." In addresses to audiences in Washington, D.C., and Australia, Westling had claimed that the learning disabilities movement cripples allegedly disabled students who could overcome their academic difficulties "with concentrated effort," demoralizes nondisabled students who recognize hoaxes performed by their peers, and "wreak[s] educational havoc," according to court documents.

The judge went on to say, "Even though Westling has referred to students with learning disabilities as 'draft dodgers' and has repeatedly voiced his concern that students without established learning disorders might be faking a disability to gain an educational advantage, to date, there has not been a single documented instance at BU in which a student has been found to have fabricated a learning disorder in order to claim eligibility for accommodations." Westling's assistant Craig Klafter was on record, the judge noted, as being equally hostile to LD students and had expressed concern about those who might be "faking" a learning disorder to get special accommodations. Remarking that mostly "rich kids have diagnoses of learning disorders," Klafter questioned whether the diagnoses where genuine. Licensed learning-disabilities specialists were, in his opinion, "snake-oil salesmen" (Guckenberger 1997).

The Boston University administrators' words and attitudes, as jarring as they are, in fact reflect the private opinions of countless Americans, including many educators. By going public with their views, Westling and Klafter (like the turncoat buddy who joined the pack in calling Dan a dummy) unwittingly did a service to the cause of LD by blasting loose hidden biases and bringing them to the surface for inspection.

No one has done more to plant and water those biases than the guru of whole language himself, Kenneth Goodman. In his 1986 monograph, which lays out the basic tenets of whole language for parents and classroom teachers, he pooh-poohs the biological glitch that hinders the acquisition of print. In a list of practices and beliefs that whole language "firmly rejects," Goodman includes this item: "believing there are substantial numbers of learners who have difficulty learning to read or write for any physical or intellectual reason" (34).

Under the heading, "Severely Labeled Children," Goodman writes, "Readers are labeled remedial, disabled, or dyslexic if they don't do well in tests and technologized [*sic*] reading programs. . . . What they suffer from most is the fact of being labeled" (36). His solution for troubled readers: "If those pupils are to become literate, they must lose their loser mentality" (56).

The strengths of these "severely labeled pupils," he says, "have been hidden by the heavy layer of their own defeatism, brought on by inappropriate over-use of word-attack skills. But it will take time. The scars are deep; the effect of years of pathological treatment and remediation will not wear off easily" (57).

Goodman does have one thing right: For kids who haven't learned to read by the time they leave grade 3, the scars are indeed deep. But as one study shows, the thing that causes trauma for LD kids—academics—is the very thing that can relieve their emotional distress. As Berninger reports, "Weiss, Catron, Harris, and Phung (1999) showed that traditional psychotherapy was no more effective than academic instruction in changing mental health status. This finding implies that fostering academic learning may have positive effects on social and emotional development" (2006).

And, as Goodman also notes correctly, solutions will take time. The older the child, the number of hours required to make him a reader grows exponen-tially. Here's what Lyon told Congress: "Unless children are identified and provided with appropriate interventions by the second or third grade, their chances of 'catching up' in reading are reduced dramatically. This does not mean that we cannot succeed with older students. We can, but the cost in both time and money is essentially tripled" (2000). So the damage done by waiting is not only emotionally enormous for the child, it is financially astronomical for the school.

That is, if the school actually intervenes effectively. If not, the costs in lost human potential are immeasurable. Of the 10 percent to 15 percent of chil-dren who eventually drop out of school, more than 75 percent will report difficulties learning to read, Lyon noted in a 2003 essay in *Perspectives*, a publication of the International Dyslexia Association. Equally startling is the fact that of students receiving special ed or compensatory education (such as Title I) for reading difficulties, a paltry 2 percent will complete a four-year college program.

Despite the steepness of the climb and the cost, nonreaders *can* be rescued at any age. "Never let it be said," wrote New York reading specialist Mary L. Burkhardt in the foreword to Flesch's 1981 book, *Why Johnny Still Can't Read*, "that if students have not learned to read by the time they are in high school, they will never learn. While it is more difficult to correct a reading problem that has existed for so long, such students should not be considered to be poor readers for years to come. Exceptional instruction and programs can correct almost all reading disabilities" (xxi).

But the science-based interventions that are scarce for young children are even more rare as kids get older. As Berninger points out, "Many schools provide explicit instruction for dyslexics when they are in the early grades, but not in middle school and high school when they would benefit from systematic, explicit language arts instruction that prepares them for the reading and writing requirements across the curriculum, study skills, note taking, and test taking" (2006).

Berninger tells the story of an eighth-grader named Sam who, because of a verbal IQ in the "very superior range," was able to pass the state's high-stakes writing test—and was then being penalized, in a sense, by being booted out of special ed, even though he struggles mightily with reading and writing. The D average he was earning was deemed "satisfactory progress" by the school. Besides, Sam has the annoying habits of asking "too many questions" and, from time to time, blurting out answers without raising his hand. These traits, which some might think are indicative of a lively mind, have gotten him into so much hot water with teachers that the school is recommending sidelining him in a program for kids with behavioral disabilities. When Sam's parents protested, Berninger reports, special-ed officials advised them to either accept the decision, or "hire a lawyer and go to a court hearing" (2006).

If a reading-disabled child has managed to finagle her way through early-grade texts by memorizing words, guessing from context, and pretending to read during SSR, her house of cards will start to crumble in grade 4. That's when kids have to start using their reading skills to gain information that is increasingly complex, unfamiliar, and technical. As Chall found in one study, "When there was too great a gap between the students' word recognition skills and the difficulty of the reading materials they were required to read, their ability to use context was no longer adequate to meet the demands" (Chall, Jacobs, and Baldwin 1990, 42–43). Shaywitz expands on this point convincingly:

> Even some children whom one might assume do not need early assessment and monitoring should have it just the same. Some especially bright children, for example, may learn to read early and seem to leapfrog over learning phonological skills. These children memorize lots of words with seeming ease and quickly build a large reading vocabulary. They simply memorize words without learning how to analyze them and pull them apart, let alone figure out how to pronounce a new or unfamiliar word. Invariably, there comes a time when such children cannot decipher the insides of these new, relatively long words—especially technical names, as in the sciences (bicarbonate, polynomial, stegosaurus), or names of people or places in history or around the world (Picasso, Lafayette, Laramie, Timbuktu, Katmandu). They have no strategy to deal with them. (2003, 196)

One analysis showed that students encountered more than 88,000 "distinct" words in school texts through ninth grade. And about half of these words—words such as inflate, extinguish, and nettle—occur only once in a billion words of text or less, making knowledge of word-formation processes an essential skill as students get older, according to William Nagy and Richard C. Anderson (1984).

But word-level decoding skills, by themselves, will not suffice. Struggling readers also need instruction designed for growth in reading—braiding word skills with guided practice in vocabulary, fluency, and comprehension—in order to achieve success in secondary school and beyond.

In a 2004 report to the Carnegie Corporation, a panel of experts addressed the complex constellation of skills that comprise mature reading. In contrast to Goodman's hey-this-reading-stuff-is-a-snap attitude, the panel recommended that schools include a rich mix of components in upper-grade reading programs. The panel's "Fifteen Elements of Effective Adolescent Literacy Programs" are: (1) direct, explicit comprehension instruction; (2) effective instructional principles embedding in content; (3) motivation and self-directed learning; (4) text-based collaborative learning; (5) strategic tutoring; (6) diverse texts; (7) intensive writing; (8) a technology component; (9) ongoing formative assessment of students; (10) extended time for literacy; (11) professional development; (12) ongoing summative assessment of students and programs; (13) teacher teams; (14) leadership; and (15) a comprehensive and coordinated literacy program.

In the Carnegie report *Reading Next: A Vision for Action and Research in Middle and High School Literacy*, authors Gina Biancarosa and Catherine Snow, both of Harvard University, issue a challenge to funders, researchers, policymakers, administrators, teachers, parents, and students to "join forces as common stakeholders" to improve the literacy of America's adolescents.

"We all hold a stake in the literacy achievement of youth, and if we do not rise to meet this challenge today, we risk our cadre of struggling readers and writers facing a future of sharply diminishing opportunities," write Biancarosa and Snow (who also served as chair of the Committee on the Prevention of Reading Difficulties in Young Children). "The ultimate beneficiaries will be not only those young people currently struggling against literacy obstacles, but also the young people of the future whose obstacles will be all the greater if we do not act now" (2004, 31).

"DYLEXIA IS ABSOLUTELY UNRELATED TO IQ"

On the day a third-grader named Matt sat down for his first private lesson in sounds and letters, Kay Kaplan's career had, in a sense, come full circle. This little boy—who couldn't read a single word despite doing first grade twice—

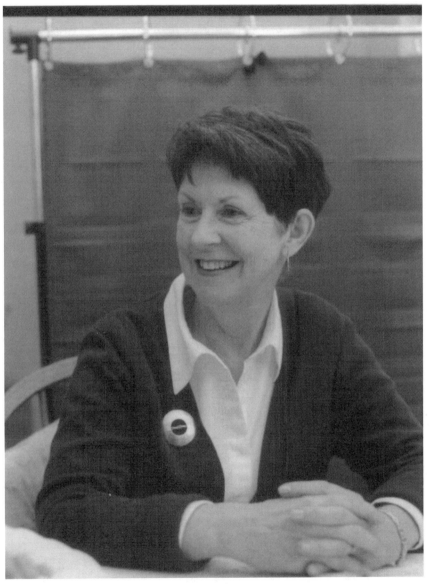

Kay Kaplan

had, quite unexpectedly, brought her back to the professional goal she cherished, but lost, some twenty years before: to teach gifted children.

Matt had an IQ that hovered in the rarified realm of genius. But his brilliant brain wasn't wired for the printed word. After two decades of work with dyslexic children, Kaplan knew just what to do to help this child fulfill his huge potential. But there was a time when she hadn't known what to do.

Her first assignment in a "really bad district" in New York was to teach language arts to the lowest-performing eighth-graders—the "bottom of the barrel," Kaplan recalls. The staff called them the "eight/nines," a reference to their abysmal reading levels on standardized tests (eighth-graders scoring at Level 9, the lowest).

"Here I was, ready to teach plot, and most of these kids were at the first- and second-grade reading level," Kaplan says, sipping tea as she reminisces in the English Tudor home she shares with her biophysicist husband in Old Portland. "I had no clue what to do. They couldn't spell, they couldn't write, they didn't know the alphabet, so they couldn't even put the spelling words in alphabetical order."

After a few months of frustration, she rummaged through her students' records looking for clues. What she found stunned her: The worst readers and spellers in the bunch had the highest IQs—normal and above.

But it wasn't until she returned to her hometown of Portland a few years later that she finally, serendipitously, came upon an answer to the enigma. She heard about a teacher named Dorothy Whitehead in the Beaverton School District who was getting great results with LD kids using a method called Orton-Gillingham. After volunteering at the school for a year, Kaplan joined Language Skills Therapy, a Portland-based group of professional tutors founded by Whitehead. Today, Kaplan coordinates the nonprofit organization—the first of its kind in the country—which employs twenty-five tutors.

When Matt's frantic parents found Kaplan, the child was enrolled in the Talented and Gifted program at one of Portland's top elementary schools. Yet the third-grader's only literacy skill was the ability to write his name. Under Kaplan's tutelage, he "just soaked it up—he was like a sponge," she recalls. In fifth grade, despite being unable to memorize his times tables, Matt got the school's highest math score on the district standardized test. "He could read the math problem and look at the four possible answers," she says. "His reasoning was so good that he could just estimate what it was."

Matt earned straight As in middle and high school, and went on to graduate summa cum laude from California Maritime Academy in Vallejo, where the boy who couldn't memorize his times tables not only received an award in math but was voted "most likely to succeed in marine architecture."

Kaplan ran into Matt's mom and dad not long ago. Her face lights up when she shares their news; to her, it feels pretty personal. "Matt," she says, "wants to teach." Sitting in her elegant blue-and-white living room, surrounded by the Japanese art she collects, Kaplan tells the story of the career she has dedicated to dyslexic kids.

Q: What did you do in those early days to try to help the "eight/nines"?

KAPLAN: I went to the reading specialist in the district and asked her about them, and she said, "Oh, they come from bad homes or they're not very smart." She just basically dismissed them. About January, I looked up the IQs of these fifteen kids—they were all boys—and it was an epiphany. It was this life-changing event, because what I discovered was that my two star students—the ones who read the best and wrote the best and spelled the best—were in the 80 range for IQ. And the worst students had average or above average IQs—in some cases, quite high.

Q: What did you do then?

KAPLAN: I went back to visit the reading expert and tossed this information at her, and she looked at me as if I were totally crazy—as if to say, "What are you talking about?" I was trying to get her to explain what this meant—why is it that the lowest-ability kids were the best readers? She just absolutely blew me off. But it was the question that stuck with me from then on.

Q: So you felt that the school was making no effort to understand or help these kids?

KAPLAN: I had a boy in my eight/nine class named Dennis. He was one of the better-behaved little boys in the class, and I liked Dennis. One day, some of the other teachers were sitting in the teachers' lounge talking about the eight/nines—one of the teachers had them for social studies and one had them for math. They were talking about what a sorry lot they were, and they said something mean about Dennis. I said something in his defense, and they said, "Well, he's a vegetable." I was so, so horrified. And they said, "Well, have you gotten any work from Dennis—anything besides a piece of paper with his name at the top?" I had to admit that I hadn't. So a couple of days later, I had the students write paragraphs—a description of a place they loved. I parked myself right beside Dennis. He had written his name at the top of his paper, and that's all. I said, "It's really hard, isn't it?" He said, "I can't." I said something about writer's block. He said, "No, I can't do it." Finally, I said, "Dennis, you mean you literally don't know how to write?" He said, "No." He was in the eighth grade. So I said, "You tell me what to write, and I'll write it down for you." So he said: "I love to go fishing. I love the

feel of the moist earth under my feet." That was not the work of a vegetable. I said, "Dennis, that's really descriptive! You're a poet!" A big
smile came over his face. I taught for a few more years in New York and
then in California, and I kept running into kids with the same syndrome—kids with a similar kind of profile. I just kept trying to figure
them out.

Q: Had you received any training in college about dealing with learning
disabilities?

KAPLAN: When I was in school for my education degree, I was specifically told there is no such thing as a learning disability. They called it a
"wastebasket" term.

Q: And then you found Dorothy Whitehead.

KAPLAN: Dorothy had adapted the Orton-Gillingham method—this great
system for teaching LD kids—for use by volunteers. As part of the training, I worked with a little boy named Danny for a year. It worked. He
learned to read. It was such a wonderful thing finally to have a technique
that would actually help these kids instead of just keeping them busy.

Q: But the teachers you ran into in New York, at least, didn't believe that
these kids could learn.

KAPLAN: Very often, teachers don't have a good working definition of
what dyslexia means. Often, they think the kids just aren't very bright—
even though dyslexia is absolutely unrelated to IQ. I've worked with
dyslexic kids who have an IQ of 135, and I've worked with dyslexic kids
who have an IQ of 80. There's no connection. Yet, many teachers see
these kids as just being "low," period.

Q: And the kids tend to buy into this perception of themselves, right?

KAPLAN: What they think is that they're dumb. They tend to generalize
their problem. It's often a huge leap for them if you can actually put a
name on it and say, "These are the things that will probably cause you
problems—for example, reading, writing, spelling. But in the other
things—creativity, problem solving, thinking—you're probably better at
it than most of the rest of us." You can honestly say that to them.

Q: What should schools be doing to catch these kids before they fail?

KAPLAN: In the ideal world, schools test kids for phonemic awareness in
kindergarten, and then get a highly phonemic reading program that is
tiered. If kids have problems, they get special help, up to and including
private tutoring in a method like Orton-Gillingham or Alphabetic Phonics or Slingerland, one-to-one, if necessary. If we did this, we would
save huge amounts of money. I look at the money the school district has
spent on special education for students I tutor—thousands and thousands

of dollars a year—and in many cases, if the school had done the appropriate thing in first grade, they wouldn't even qualify for special ed.

Q: Why do so many teachers reject the findings of research coming out of the National Institutes of Health or the National Reading Panel?

KAPLAN: These findings, which support direct instruction in phonics, are the exact opposite of what most teachers have been taught to do. The whole-language movement that came in like a tidal wave several decades ago argues that because all normal children learn to talk by being in a rich environment of language, all children will learn to read and write in exactly the same way. You just surround them with wonderful literature. Because of this wonderful brain that these children have, this wonderful capacity for language, they will automatically learn to read and write. Many good things came out of this belief—"language experience," for example, where kids in kindergarten would tell you stories and you would write them down. Instead of these boring, dull phonics pages, there was a rocking chair and pillows and the carpet and the Big Books. And you had "guess-and-go" spelling. All of that is terrific. Kids with good visual memory for words and kids on the top end of the scale for grasping the phonemic code took off. But the other kids who were often just as bright—or even way brighter—who had weak visual memory for symbols and could not attach letters to the code were dead in the water. Still, people kept saying, "They'll get it—it's developmental, just like speech." I probably would have bought the whole-language thing had I not met the eight/nines. Because of those kids, I absolutely knew it wasn't true.

"THESE SIXTH-GRADERS CAN'T READ A LICK"

Hell-bent on discovery, Danny Tibbetts couldn't wait to ditch his books and head out after school. Lying on his stomach in the reedy marsh near his suburban home, the little boy learned firsthand about the habitat and life cycle of frogs. Tinkering in the dusty half-light of the garage, he uncovered the inner workings of small engines. Scavenging scraps of wood and metal, he designed and built all sorts of wheeled rigs powered by batteries and imagination. Those were his happy hours.

His classroom hours, however, were agonizing. Danny got off to a bad start, failing to nail down his ABCs and having to repeat kindergarten. Things never got much better. After years of pullout remediation and private tutoring, he gained the ability to decode words up to a third-grade level. But when

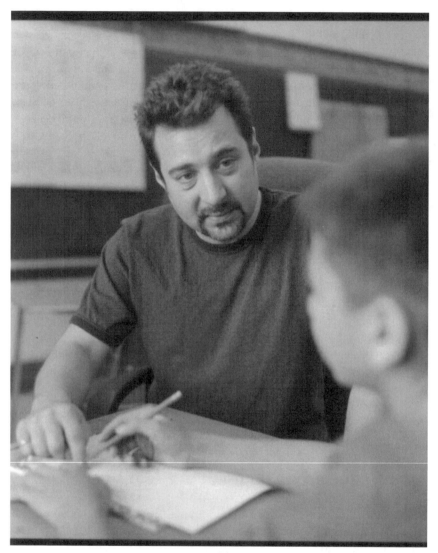

Dan Tibbetts

he left high school at age eighteen without a diploma, he still couldn't read for comprehension.

Danny's story, however, doesn't end with a low-wage job at a car wash or pizza parlor. This most unlikely candidate for college, deeply determined not to be "a loser," eventually made his way to the university. And the boy who couldn't decipher even the most basic basal readers ended up in the most unlikely of places—back in the public school classroom. This time, though, he stands at the front of a class full of kids he understands as well as he understands himself. That's because, like him, his students in the Intensive Learning Center at Portland's Beaumont Middle School are all learning disabled.

"These kids often come in at the first-grade level, across the board, in their language arts skills," says Dan Tibbetts, catching a brief respite at his desk while his twelve students labor over sentence construction. "They can't read a lick, they can't write a lick. Somehow, they got to sixth grade. They should have been in a program like this a long time ago."

The "program like this" blends direct instruction in the skills of reading and writing—beginning with the fundamental building blocks of letter recognition and phonemic awareness—with lots of behavior management and one-to-one attention. The curriculum draws on the very strategies that turned things around for Tibbetts when, at age nineteen, he enrolled in a program at Portland Community College for nonreading adults. "The curriculum was based on Corrective Reading from Science Research Associates," he says. "Boy, that's when things really picked up for me."

Once the trick to reading clicked in, Tibbetts became a committed bibliophile. Now forty, he pores voraciously over print materials of all kinds, particularly biography, philosophy, and current events—with a special love for the history of rock 'n' roll. At Beaumont Middle School, he passes on his hard-won wisdom to his emotionally bruised LD students. One parent whose child was in Tibbetts's class wrote this to district administrators: "The difference this program has made in my son's life is beyond measure. In one year, he has gone from terrified to triumphant."

Another parent said: "Prior to the ILC, our son was beginning to lose his self-confidence, feeling overwhelmed by school demands and beginning to believe that he was stupid. To see him beginning to fall apart was very difficult for us. Dan Tibbetts has helped our son reestablish the confidence he once had by providing an appropriate curriculum that really works, implementing it in a way that enabled him to succeed in areas he found impossible, and providing the care and support of a safe and enriching learning environment. I will walk, send letters and e-mails, give speeches, carry banners, contact anybody and everybody to assure a future for and expansion of these classes."

Q: Do you remember how you felt as a young child who couldn't master reading skills?

TIBBETTS: Oh, man, it was so tough on me, and pretty rough on my parents. I was hurt by the whole thing. Kids teased me, so I acted out. I was very goofy. I liked getting attention for being funny. I got in trouble for everything—it didn't matter what class I was in. I couldn't memorize; I couldn't recite the flag salute. I got in trouble for not paying attention. I got spankings from the principal. Psychologists call these negative behaviors that LD kids get caught up in "schemas." They're scripts—built-in programs that come back and play out under stress.

Q: What strategies were tried for helping you learn?

TIBBETTS: I had all the bells and whistles growing up as an LD kid. By my third-grade year, my parents got me a tutor. In fourth grade, I got into the Chapter 1 reading program.

Q: Why didn't the resource room approach work for you?

TIBBETTS: Kids who have darn-near grade-level skills and just need someone to help them close that little gap in their regular schoolwork need a resource teacher to help them achieve their mainstream goals. But when you have a kid who's several years behind, he or she can't keep up, no matter what, in that regular classroom. Full inclusion is ineffective for remediating basic skills deficits. I can tell you that when kids are way behind in their skills in reading and writing and general knowledge, they're not going to be able to keep up with their average peers. It's embarrassing and frustrating for everyone—the student, the teacher, the parents. Students with severe learning disabilities nearly always require intensive individual or small-group instruction for at least a portion of the day.

Q: You didn't earn a high school diploma, yet you went to college. How did that happen?

TIBBETTS: When high school was over, I had this sense that, "Man, I don't want to be a loser." I knew the first thing I had to do was learn to read. So one day when I was nineteen, I got together with my aunt, who's a teacher, and my dad, and I said, "I can't read." My aunt had a friend at Lewis & Clark College, an instructor in the school psychology program, who evaluated me and diagnosed my learning disability. She steered me to Portland Community College, where they had a specialist who was teaching LD students to read, write, and spell. I learned all of the phonemes from scratch. I worked hard at it—man, I worked really hard. They met with you every week, they phoned you, they helped you get the credits you needed. And, wow, things just really started turning and really cruised for me. I became independent very quickly, within a year. I always made sure I got an A or a B. I got enough credits to go to a four-year university.

Q: Where did you go to college?

TIBBETTS: I went to Southern Oregon College (now Southern Oregon

State University). It was in the early, early '80s. I was one of the first LD adults to get to college and have advocacy behind me. With my documented learning disability, I got accommodations under IDEA—extra time for tests and assignments, more attention from instructors. Meanwhile, the university started up a student disability union—back then, they called it Handicapped Student Services. I was hired to assist the director. I didn't know anything about computers when I started, but I helped put together a computer lab with Commodore 64s and in the process learned to use the computer. That's what really helped me get through college.

Q: Why is direct instruction so unpopular among many educators?

TIBBETTS: It's dry. But it works. It's a method of disciplined instruction based on mastery learning. You don't go on to Step 2 till you've mastered Step 1. You start at the student's skill level, correct errors right away, review as you go along, and fill in any gaps. It builds a real strong foundation.

Q: What do you like best about working with LD kids?

TIBBETTS: I get my rewards by seeing the little, teeny bits of progress that kids make each day turn into big progress over time. Using this approach, and using it right, I've almost never had a kid who hasn't made good progress.

"THERE ARE A FEW CURMUDGEONS IN EVERY INSTITUTION"

Dale Holloway was running late on the afternoon of our scheduled interview. Midterm exams and papers were looming at Lewis & Clark College, where Holloway coordinates services for disabled students, and she'd been deeply involved in a discussion with a dyslexic freshman who was struggling to convert the knowledge in her head into prose on paper. Immersed in the challenge of helping the student express the philosophical nuances of Locke, Rousseau, Hobbes, and Plato—readings in the "Inventing America" freshman course—Holloway suddenly noticed the time and grabbed her tote bag. Rushing out the door, she promised to pick up the discussion again the next day—right after meeting with a dyslexic sophomore who needed some coaching on his sociology course work. Both of these students, she tells us when she finally arrives, are typical of the hundreds of learning-disabled college students she has worked with over the years. "They tend to be holistic thinkers, not linear thinkers," she says. "But they have to do linear thinking for school."

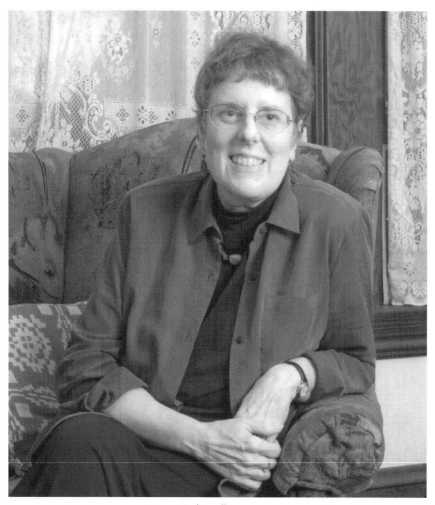

Dale Holloway

The private, liberal arts college—set serenely among wild tangles of mosses and ferns in Portland's wooded West Hills—originally hired Holloway as a writing coach. She was only vaguely aware of dyslexia back then. But she soon noticed a pattern of learning problems among certain students who came to the Writing Center for help. She was curious. She started stopping by the library after work, browsing the stacks, looking for insights. Before she knew it, she had segued from part-time writing instructor to round-the-clock expert on learning disabilities. Today, she oversees services for about 150 disabled students (mostly LD, but including some deaf, blind, and physically limited students) and also runs the Reversals support group that has given information, encouragement, and advice to hundreds of parents and students during the nineteen years since she founded it.

Q: What prompted your switch from writing coach to coordinator of services for disabled students?

HOLLOWAY: As a writing instructor, I had always adhered to the school of thought that said, "If a student is writing unclear prose, his or her thinking is unclear." Yet when I was working in the Writing Center helping students with their papers, I began to notice that certain students didn't fit that pattern. They were very, very bright and they were thinking very clearly, but they just weren't converting those thoughts into the right words. They tended to be very holistic thinkers, but they'd leave out important pieces of information when they were writing essays. They usually had spelling problems and punctuation problems. Eventually, I found out that one of these students had been diagnosed as dyslexic. So I started reading up on dyslexia, and I went to an International Dyslexia Association conference in Seattle. It was an eye-opener.

Q: What did you do with your new information?

HOLLOWAY: I came back and started a support group for these kids, because they had a whole lot of anxiety around writing. Then I persuaded the administration to let me teach a class for them, working on writing and reading skills, study skills, organizational skills. There were just seven or eight students and they loved meeting together, but they didn't want anybody else on campus to know why they were meeting. So we always had to find a room with no windows for our meeting.

Q: How do kids with learning disabilities get to college in the first place if they were never identified or given special help in their early years?

HOLLOWAY: They're bright kids. They figure out the system. I think many of them learn to read well enough to fake it. They may actually think they're reading well, even when they're not. They're recognizing words by shape, and they're bright enough to guess a lot of words from context. They pick up a lot in class, and they talk with their friends as a way to absorb the material.

Q: So they get admitted, and then things start to unravel?

HOLLOWAY: They come to college, and they're suddenly faced with an enormous amount of reading. In high school, they could compensate for their reading problems by spending more time than other kids on their studies. But in college, there just aren't enough hours in a day to compensate for all the reading they're assigned. Their foreign language class

moves so much faster than it did in high school. They just can't handle
it. They hit a wall. That's when they wind up in my office, and we advise
them to get tested for learning disabilities.

Q: What kinds of accommodations can LD students get at Lewis & Clark
through your office?

HOLLOWAY: We provide note-takers, books-on-tape, tutors. We advocate
for extra time on exams, and we have separate rooms for testing for students who have attention issues or anxiety issues. We offer proofreaders
for dyslexic students to go over the next-to-the-last draft and help them
fix the punctuation and spelling. We might provide a coach if the student
has problems with organization or attention. There's nothing scarier for
somebody with an attention deficit disorder than to be looking at a four-
month project. If there's a big paper due, we'll hire another student to
be a "thesis buddy" to walk them through the whole process—to meet
with them once a week, set goals for the week, read what they've written, give them feedback, set goals for the following week.

Q: What sorts of one-to-one supports do you, personally, offer to LD students?

HOLLOWAY: One of the most comprehensive things I do is advising about
classes to take—helping them balance their class load. A lot of what I do
is strategic planning with the students—really strategizing around their
learning style. The student's regular advisor says, "You need to take the
following three classes for your major." And then the student comes to
me, and I'll say, "OK, but don't take these two classes during the same
semester. It's too much reading all at once, or each of those classes
requires a huge research paper." I also advocate with the financial aid
office for students who need to take reduced course loads and so will
need more time to get their degree. I also coach a lot of students personally. I have a number of ADD students who meet with me for half an
hour each week to check in—how did things go last week, what's coming up next week? If something's sliding, we figure out how to fix it.

Q: Where does the funding for all these services come from?

HOLLOWAY: From the college budget. That's one of the big differences
between K–12 and higher ed—there's no federal funding for accommodations at the college level.

Q: Is the faculty supportive of these kinds of accommodations?

HOLLOWAY: Overall, yes. Our higher administration has been adamant
about obeying the law and has been supportive of me. Most teachers are
great about it. Right now, we're in midterms and we have all sorts of
faculty who are sending copies of their exams to us so that we can test
the students in our office. Many of our teachers now put a note on their

course syllabus that says, "If you have a disability, please let me know and then go to Student Support Services." Many of them, especially the younger ones, are very matter-of-fact about learning differences. They'll discuss it with the student in a very straightforward way, and so it's not stigmatized at all.

Q: Do you ever run into resistance or negativity from the faculty?

HOLLOWAY: Once in a while. There are a few individual faculty members who feel that some of their goals are being compromised by providing an accommodation, and then we usually have a discussion about that—do the course goals, for instance, really involve speed? Some teachers feel that it's really important for the student to do this work very fast. We examine that assumption, and then try to come up with some kind of compromise. There are always a few curmudgeons. A couple of faculty members have refused to give students extra time on exams because the students were doing well in their class. The assumption is that only people who don't do well in classes—people who aren't "smart"—need accommodations. We have a growing body of scientific evidence to show that it's possible, for instance, to have a 135 IQ yet have a processing speed that's at the 9th percentile. Or that it's possible to have a brilliant verbal IQ and still not be able to spell every third word. But there are still these pockets of resistance, and some skepticism about the whole nature of learning disability.

Q: Do the laws that cover college students differ from the laws that cover K–12 students?

HOLLOWAY: K–12 is governed by IDEA, while higher ed is still under the old Rehabilitation Act of 1973, Section 504. Mainly, we're charged with enforcing 504. The attention given to the 1990 Americans with Disabilities Act seemed to give 504 a lot more teeth—it empowered us a whole lot more. One of the main differences is that under IDEA, the schools have the responsibility for identifying disabilities and providing services, whether the students ask for them or not. At the college level, students are viewed as adults, and they have to request the accommodations. Colleges also require documentation for services—a battery of cognitive tests and an achievement battery. It's a pretty hefty bit of documentation.

Q: Does research show evidence of how accommodations impact student performance?

HOLLOWAY: A number of researchers now have duplicated the 1991 research by M. Kay Runyan of UC-Berkeley showing that if you give non-learning-disabled students extended time on exams they do a little bit better, but not significantly better. But if you give learning-disabled students extra time, they do *significantly* better. I flash those charts all the time when I talk to faculty, because it shows a qualitative difference in the way somebody with a learning disability takes in and gives out information.

Q: Do the services you provide make a difference in your students' academic careers?

HOLLOWAY: We did a study in the late '80s in which we divided disabled students as to whether or not they used accommodations and services, and then looked at their college careers. Those who used the services actually had a higher GPA than the average Lewis & Clark student, and their retention rate was higher than the retention rate for the college as a whole. Those disabled students who didn't use the services had a retention rate that was below the average.

Q: What happens to these LD students once they get out into the workplace?

HOLLOWAY: We had a student with a social science degree who was working in a group home. She had to write up case notes every night. When she started, she asked if she could dictate the notes and have them transcribed, and they said no. So she had to haul these things home and kill herself every night writing them up. But she was so good in her position that pretty soon they asked her to manage the whole house. She said, "Well, I'm sorry, I can't do that if I have to write up all these notes; it would be impossible." They said, "That's fine—you can dictate them, and we'll give you a transcriber." There have been a lot of cases like that, where if they can prove themselves in one area, their employer is much more willing to provide accommodations in another.

Q: Do you have another example?

HOLLOWAY: We had a student several years back who was so dyslexic that she would write entire ten-page papers without using a single piece of punctuation. She worked in my office, but she wasn't allowed to file because she didn't know the alphabet. She took German and I was a nervous wreck the whole time, but she made it through with very, very hard work. She was brilliant. She was a real strategist, a really good thinker and problem solver. Once her teachers got over her spelling on exams, they realized how brilliant she was and recognized her analytical ability. She headed up a group that pushed for some changes on campus in a very diplomatic and reasonable way. She graduated Phi Beta Kappa with honors in international affairs.

Q: What happened after she graduated?

HOLLOWAY: She got an internship at an aerospace firm in Iowa as a policy strategist. She was wonderful at doing research and she could express complex ideas really well, orally. She'd make presentations to the engineers at this Iowa firm, based on the research she did. They would then decide which directions they wanted to move in based on those strategizing meetings. Then, believe it or not, she landed a similar job at an aerospace firm in Germany, and later went on to France. Now, she's back in the States and she's in grad school at a prestigious university studying law and diplomacy.

Q: She must have had a great support structure at home.

HOLLOWAY: Her mother had spent most of her childhood reading all of her schoolbooks to her. When she was in middle school, she decided she didn't want her mother reading her schoolbooks to her for the rest of her life, so she learned to read her books to herself out loud—that was the only way she could do it. Her major was a field that required a huge amount of reading. I took her to a conference with me once, and we shared a room. She said, "Do you mind if I read out loud?" And I said, "No, go right ahead." She would read a paragraph, and then she would go back and she'd reread selected sentences as she underlined them. Then she'd kind of mutter to herself—I think trying to consolidate information—and then move on to the next paragraph. This went on for hours and hours and hours. That's how she got herself through college.

Q: And she is not an exception in being successful after college?

HOLLOWAY: Oh, no. Many of our other students are really good at computers, developing and designing websites. A couple of them gained and lost gobs of money during the dot-com era of the late '90s. We have some who are very involved in environmental activities and environmental businesses. A number of them are teachers—better teachers, in fact, than their own teachers were. A number of them are artists. Many of them are in social work, some are physical therapists, a couple of them are doctors. I just talked to one former student who has his MD and PhD and is doing research in London on important diseases.

"MOST IEPS ARE USELESS"

It seemed a little bit incongruous, meeting one of the nation's leading experts in special-ed law at a truck stop. But when University of Oregon emeritus professor Barbara Bateman pulled into the parking lot with her dog Mister Binkster riding shotgun and then strode up to the counter at TJ's wearing a pair of well-worn jeans and a plaid shirt, she looked like she could be a regular.

Bateman's residence outside the quiet Oregon village of Creswell is, however, only a jumping-off point for her legal consulting practice—and, not incidentally, her wildlife adventuring. One week, she'll leave the filbert orchards, Marionberry fields, and grass-seed silos of the Willamette Valley to confer with a legal team in Philadelphia (or Honolulu or Orlando or Austin or Sitka, Alaska) over the educational rights of autistic or dyslexic kids. The next week, she's packing her snorkeling gear for a shelling expedition in the Sea of Cortez with one of the world's leading conchologists.

Her "Number One fun thing" to do, though, is birding. Bateman's is not the tame version of watching birds—the binoculars-in-the-domestic-woodlands approach. Hers is an extreme sport—the digiscope-in-the-international-hinterlands style of birding. She has stalked the lilac-breasted roller through the savannas of East Africa. She has followed the call of the improbable three-wattled bellbird for hours through the Costa Rican rain forest, and crouched in the marshlands of Trinidad, straining for a glimpse of the scarlet ibis. "Don't get me started talking about birds," she cautions, as she warms to the subject. The implication: You might be here all day.

The other topic she can talk about all day is special education. The author of dozens of articles and a shelf-full of books on the legal and practical aspects of interpreting and using the Individuals with Disabilities Education Act, Bateman uses direct language that sometimes has an in-your-face tone when she voices her frustrations about getting schools to comply not only with the letter of the law, but also the spirit. Not prone to weasel words or prevarication, Bateman calls a crock a crock. In the article "Writing Individualized Education Programs (IEPs) for Success" posted on the special-ed advocacy website Wrightslaw, for instance, she makes the provocative statement, "Most IEPs are useless—or slightly worse." We asked her to elaborate.

Q: How could an IEP actually be *worse* than useless?
BATEMAN: Worse than useless because it wastes time, it looks like somebody's actually doing something, and it can be sold to a naïve hearing officer as if, "Oh, look, we've got this thirty-two-page document."
Q: So it creates an illusion.
BATEMAN: Exactly. There should be a requirement that hearing officers be knowledgeable about special education. I mean, you'll get a civil engineer or a retired computer programmer, and some of them are great. They see through the crap. Others just let the crap flow over them, and they buy whatever the school people say. Absolutely, a hearing officer should have to be knowledgeable.
Q: How did you get started in the field of learning disabilities?
BATEMAN: I got into learning disabilities totally by accident. When I realized I was interested in special ed, I asked my master's advisor

where I should go for a doctorate. She said, "Wherever Sam Kirk is."
So I found him at the University of Illinois and went to study with him.
In the 1930s, Sam had studied with Marion Monroe, who wrote *Children Who Cannot Read* in 1932. Monroe was the first one to use the
idea of discrepancy (between IQ and achievement). In 1962, Sam and I
coauthored the first article to use the term he coined, "learning disabilities," in print. My office at the university was right next door to
researcher Carl Bereiter when Siegfried Engelmann was hired as a
research assistant. Zig would come into Carl's office and talk to him. If
you've ever heard Zig's voice, you'd know I had no choice but to listen
to everything he said—it carried right through the wall. So here I was—
complete chance, circumstance: Sam Kirk is my advisor, and Zig Engelmann is talking in my ear every day.

Q: What prompted your later career shift into special-ed law?

BATEMAN: My frustration was that I'd known all this stuff about how to
teach reading—and thereby reduce the numbers of so-called LD students—since 1960, and there were people around who'd known it much,
much longer than that. Yet many of our schools persisted in not doing it.
So I came to the idea that law could be a tool—or a club—to force the
schools to do it right. But my first year of law school, I learned that there
is no such thing as educational malpractice because education has no
standards against which malpractice could be judged. I was very disappointed. But by that time, I was hooked on law. When I graduated in '76,
IDEA was poised to go into effect, and there were not a lot of people at
that time with backgrounds in both law and special ed. So I went into
special-ed law instead of suing schools for not teaching reading properly.

Q: Why has the research supporting direct instruction in phonics been
rejected by so many in the educational mainstream?

BATEMAN: I've asked myself that question thousands of times. I think
it's one of the most interesting questions there is. I absolutely don't
know, but I have glimmers. One thing I have learned over the years is
that regular educators—in contrast to school-psych people, special-ed
people, research people, or any other professional group I've run up
against—tend to be "warm fuzzies." This is a generalization, of course.
But they tend to be right-brained. Data do not seem to impress them.
They go by impressions, global ideas, holistic healings. I've seen universities trying to merge special ed and regular ed. It doesn't work. It's oil
and water. It's two different breeds of cats. And I say that without any
judgment, truly.

Q: What else?

BATEMAN: The next piece *is* a little judgmental, and I don't feel comfortable about that. But when you buy into direct instruction, you buy into an accountability philosophy. You recognize that the child's learning is the responsibility of the teacher, and that if the child hasn't learned it's because he or she wasn't adequately taught. There is still that possibility that the kid really has some kind of brain glitch that makes it much more difficult. But I think there's a fear of accountability. When you buy into a whole-language philosophy where you're letting the child "blossom" into reading and all you're doing is "fertilizing" or "sprinkling" or whatever the heck they're doing, you're sidestepping the accountability issue because learning is up to the child and the print-rich environment—it's not the direct function of the teacher. This sidestepping accountability may be related to the right-brain, warm-fuzzy nurturance. Those are only two little pieces of the big mystery.

Q: Many educators argue that if parents don't introduce their child to literacy at home, then schools really can't be held responsible when the child doesn't learn to read.

BATEMAN: Which Engelmann and others of his expertise have proven is just a crock. You can teach kids in spite of any and all of those things, if you know how to do it.

Q: What is the school's responsibility, under the law, to identify and serve kids with learning disabilities?

BATEMAN: First, the school has to find all the kids. The "Child Find" requirement of IDEA is a major responsibility squarely on the school. Then, for each individual child, the school has to do a "full and individual evaluation in all areas related to the suspected disability." Then the law says that the school will develop an "individualized education program" that contains the services needed to address all of the child's unique educational needs. The law is fine. The problem is that school people don't do it.

Q: Which leaves it in the lap of the parents.

BATEMAN: Parents are the only ones who really have the legal authority, the power, to go after the school to make them do it. And yet the school is responsible for telling the parents what their rights are and how they're supposed to make this machinery work. So we have the classic case of the fox guarding the henhouse. Many schools do not share with parents any more meaningful information than they have to.

Q: How can this Catch 22 be corrected?

BATEMAN: It would help if school people themselves knew more about the law. There's an awful lot of ignorance out there, as opposed to bad faith. A lot school people just truly don't know. But there are also a lot who *do* know and very carefully don't do one bit more than the parents compel them to do. Very few parents know how to do that.

Q: You write that parents' route to getting the appropriate education for their child is to make sure the IEP team writes "measurable" goals. We don't see that happening often.

BATEMAN: I think the situation is even dimmer than you think. What we're finding is that even in that slowly increasing tiny segment of school people who *do* write measurable goals and objectives, the next battle is to get them to actually measure them. I've almost stopped talking *just* about "measurable." Now, I'm trying to link "measurable" and "measured," as if it were one great big word.

Q: How often do parents prevail against school districts in LD lawsuits?

BATEMAN: Parents almost never win in LD cases. There has been a tremendous misreading of the landmark case from 1982—*Board of Education* vs. *Rowley*—which is often cited in LD cases. That misreading has resulted in hearing officers in schools believing that methodology is solely at the discretion of the school. I believe that was a legal error from the beginning. The '97 IDEA amendments made it clear that there are times when methodology *does* have to be part of the IEP. But a lot of schools and hearing officers still don't know that, and so they just automatically say, "Oh, this is about methodology, and so the school can do whatever it wants."

Q: What's your opinion of Oregon's Portland School District going to a full-inclusion model and getting rid of programs for LD kids?

BATEMAN: Number one, it's against the law. Number two, it's against common sense. I think what Portland is doing is an absolute abomination. It is illegal.

"I SAW EXTREMELY POOR OUTCOMES FOR THESE KIDS"

If you were a kid whose life was a nightmarish mess of abuse and neglect, you couldn't hope for a better ally than Brian Baker. As an attorney with the public-interest law firm Juvenile Rights Project, Baker is a flesh-and-blood embodiment of the concept of advocacy, in both its legal and its personal senses.

The Oxford dictionary's three definitions of "advocate"—a person who supports or speaks in favor, a person who pleads for another, and a professional pleader in a court of justice—all apply to the work Baker does helping some of Oregon's most troubled children get the educational services guaran-

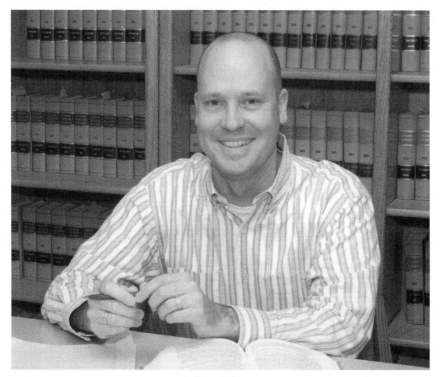

Brian Baker

teed to them under the law. Kids who wind up in the courts, either as dependents or as delinquents, are a lot more likely than other kids to have learning disabilities. But because of the chaotic circumstances of their lives, they are a lot less likely to get help for those disabilities. That's where Baker comes in. He and his colleagues at JRP step up to make sure court-involved kids learn to read and compute, finish high school, and have a fighting chance at a decent future.

Baker's knowledge of the law gets him through the convoluted red tape, the complex regulations, and the institutional resistance that so often impede children's access to special education in the public schools. But it's the fire in his gut that gets him through the wrenching sixty-hour weeks, going to bat for kids who can be simultaneously tough and vulnerable, maddening and fragile, defiant and depressed, heedless and needy. Their outward behavior tends to mirror the turbulence within. Schools, faced with dwindling resources and swelling class sizes, very often resort to punitive rather than preventive measures with troubled children—unless Baker and his colleagues happen to show up with copies of the federal Individuals with Disabilities Education Act or the Americans with Disabilities Act, Section 504, snapped into their briefcases.

Brian Baker could be making big bucks in a corporate law firm downtown. Instead, he's chosen to be a champion of children who don't have many people in their corner. When burnout threatens, Baker looks at his own children, safe and secure and loved. And then he soldiers on for the other kids.

Q: What steered you toward juvenile law?

BAKER: When I was just out of law school, I was a prosecutor working with families in domestic violence cases, and then started a general practice as a juvenile public defender. Probably 80 percent of my cases were "dependencies"—child welfare cases of abuse and neglect with court-appointed attorneys. These were kids of all ages, from one-day-old, drug-affected infants to fourteen-year-old children who'd been sexually abused and removed from their homes to twenty-one-year-olds who had developmental disabilities and were still under the protection of the system. Two to three years into that practice, I began to recognize that the systems that serve children aren't focused on education. The courts and child welfare agencies focus on protection, imminent health and safety, foster placement. But I didn't see the school piece discussed in review hearings. I didn't see it coming up in citizen review boards, which are volunteers who oversee children in substitute care. It often was left with the parent or foster parent to pursue special ed.

Q: What did you do about it?

BAKER: These children don't have a consistent, knowledgeable person to fill the role of parent or surrogate—to be an advocate. I observed very high mobility, loss of school records, delays in transfer of records. It's not uncommon for the kids to experience two, three, four moves within a school year across district boundaries. With each one of those moves, there's a substantial loss of educational progress. Records don't get transferred, identification and evaluation for special-ed services get derailed. I started to carve out a little time here and there to research the issues, to see what was happening nationally. In the last three or four years, a burst of research has come out looking at the educational circumstances of children in foster care and child welfare. Finally, folks are starting to address those issues from the research end.

Q: What steps has your firm taken to better address the educational needs of its clients?

BAKER: We started to push into more individual advocacy for our kids on the education front—making forays out to attend IEP meetings or 504 meetings, to attend disciplinary, suspension, and expulsion hearings. We developed training materials, and then hit the road to train folks connected to the child welfare and juvenile justice systems—parents, foster parents, judges, advocates, caseworkers.

Q: What kind of training do you give to parents and foster parents?

BAKER: It's mostly on special-ed advocacy and alerting them to the unique issues of our population of kids. We emphasize multidisciplinary team building, where the parent or foster parent brings together the caseworker and the mental health therapist or the development disabilities case manager—all of these systems that can bring resources to the table to support the child.

Q: Having an effective advocate is critical for kids, yet so many disadvantaged parents are unfamiliar with the law and their child's rights, or they're simply unable to take on the school system for reasons that may be cultural, logistical, or emotional. This is a huge impediment in a system that rarely works without strong parental involvement.

BAKER: A lot of overwhelmed families are struggling just to keep it together, so I do a lot of bridge building between families and schools. When breakdowns in services and communications occur, we step in and try to keep things moving forward. School administrators and teachers often say they can't serve the child because they don't have a responsive parent. But many times there's a disconnect between the school's expectation of the parents' participation and the realities of low-SES families and single-parent homes. In trainings, I offer this example: the single parent who works days and can't call the school, let alone come in, who tries to call the school at night but finds that there's no way of leaving a message, and who, even if they *could* come in at night, doesn't have child care or transportation. We're saying, how can we all start talking creatively about connecting? There are some great models out there. I like the community-school models—one-stop shopping where all kinds of services are available at the school. The school is a hub.

Q: Your website cites research showing that disabilities, including learning disabilities, are significantly more common among kids in the system, especially those in corrections.

BAKER: Generally, kids in the juvenile justice system have much higher incidences of disabilities than other kids. It's as high as three-fourths of the kids in youth corrections facilities. The most recent Oregon Youth Authority report showed about 78 percent of kids coming out of youth corrections facilities had school-based disabilities, primarily learning disabilities, emotional disturbances, or cognitive disabilities. That's very high when you compare it to the 12 percent to 13 percent in the general school-age population.

Q: By school-based disabilities, you mean anything that would get you into special ed through IDEA or disability law?

BAKER. Yes. A fairly typical situation for our clients is having both behavioral and learning disabilities—multiple disabilities—that affect school achievement.

Q: Do many of these disabilities go unidentified in the schools?

BAKER: Definitely, our kids are underidentified. Sometimes there's a lot of difficulty just getting initial evaluations going, which is interesting given how stringent the "Child Find" requirements of IDEA are. It's a huge issue. I've had cases where we've had to meet four or five times. The tension that exists in IEP meetings, I think, is the tension between individual needs versus available resources. It simply comes down to that.

Q: What should schools and social services do to be more effective in identifying school-based disabilities soon enough to prevent disastrous outcomes?

BAKER: We've got to be much better about communicating when children move or are moved, identifying liaisons and clear chains of information sharing—similar to some of the rules in place for homeless children under the McKinney-Vento Homeless Assistance Act. That legislation has set out a lot of protections for homeless children, including having a liaison at the district level whose ultimate responsibility is to problem solve and make sure that homeless children are in school, that they are enrolled immediately, that they're not kept out because records are not there.

Q: You talk about the "vicious cycle" of educational failure leading to involvement in the justice system, which in turn leads to a downward spiral for the child's life.

BAKER: Studies on our population of kids show that there are much higher rates of dropping out. Once you drop out of school, there are very poor outcomes—the need for public assistance, involvement in juvenile or adult corrections, single parenthood, substance abuse, poor nutrition. Teens with disabilities who are in foster care have more school transfers, greater likelihood of movement into alternative education, lower GPAs, less participation in statewide testing. There is a unique complex of risk factors among the kids we're working with. They don't have just one or two risk factors, but five or six risk factors, any one of which is significant in and of itself. There's also the issue of minority overrepresentation in special ed, foster care, and school discipline.

Q: How often does instructional methodology come up in IEP meetings?

BAKER: Families and advocates, as noneducators, struggle to know which methodology should be used. A significant difficulty is how we translate the IEP process and the special-ed documents into the regular-ed setting. Regular-ed teachers are part of the IEP team, but it's often difficult to get buy-in or communication between special ed and regular ed. In the worst-case scenario, I will hear that a teacher thinks the kid's lazy, or he's not trying hard enough. I think there's this "lost in translation" between special ed and regular ed. I've been to some buildings where the IEPs are not distributed to the regular-ed teachers, and the regular-ed teachers aren't taking the initiative to access them.

Q: Will you talk about the work you've done with support from the Edward J. Byrne Federal Juvenile Violence Prevention Grant, administered by the Oregon State Police?

BAKER: Under the Byrne grant, we've created a model of heightened advocacy for kids who are in the dependency or delinquency system. There has never been adequate funding, support, or guidance to juvenile-court attorneys or attorneys for children to take a look at the school piece. So we have a screening tool, and we assess every kid for attendance, achievement, and behavior within the school. If there are problems in any of those areas, we assign an attorney. We have four attorneys who have caseloads of just the school piece for our clients. Working closely with the dependency or delinquency attorney, we review school records, request assessments, request IEPs if it's appropriate. Hopefully, we're going to be able to show better achievement, less mobility, fewer behavioral issues, and try to make a pitch that this needs to be encompassed in how the state provides services and legal representation.

Q: Are you optimistic about educational opportunities for LD kids in the future?

BAKER: I was at a conference a couple of years ago and I met a very well-known juvenile psychologist who was retiring. He told me that in thirty years of practice, his greatest frustration was not being able to better bridge his individual diagnostic work with school-based services. He said we have a nineteenth-century system in a twenty-first-century world.

"WE'VE GOT TO GET SERVICES TO KIDS EARLIER"

Rousseau, a wiry mix of black Lab and red heeler, sits placidly at the feet of fourteen-year-old Kevin as the boy brushes the dog's glossy coat. Four-year-

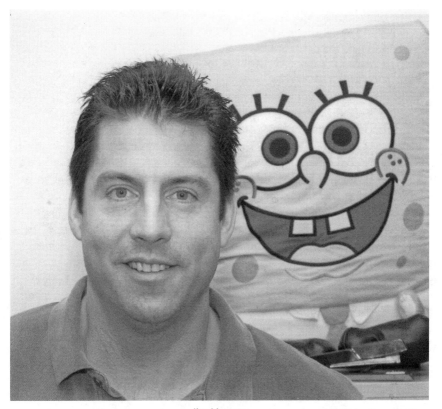

Jim Hanson

old Rousseau doesn't know he's a therapy dog. He just knows that on Fridays, he gets to hang out with his owner Jim Hanson at the Metropolitan Learning Center (MLC), where kids like Kevin come to talk about life.

When Kevin sat down for his bimonthly appointment with the school psychologist, he was talking fast and patting Rousseau with quick, staccato motions. But after picking up the dog brush and running it through Rousseau's coat for a few minutes, the rapid patting gave way to a measured cadence and a fluid motion. Kevin's speech gradually slowed down. As he relaxed, his thought processes evened out and he was able to express himself more fully. What Jason didn't realize was that brushing Rousseau wasn't really about improving the pooch's appearance, but rather about helping Hanson guide his young client toward better social adjustment.

Kevin is one of about fifteen kids with Asperger's syndrome who attend this 420-student alternative school in a gentrified section of Northwest Portland. As the lone school psychologist in a school full of students who, for one reason or another, find regular public schools a poor fit, Hanson needs every bit of assistance he can get—canine or otherwise—to keep up with the load. On alternating days, he works with special-needs students at two additional schools.

The props jammed into every niche of Hanson's narrow MLC office include a stuffed SpongeBob SquarePants character, a nearly life-size dolphin, and "Jabber Jaws"—a talking skull that repeats kids' words when they speak into its mouth. The toys help build rapport by soothing kids' fears and encouraging conversation, he explains.

Working with children is, for Hanson, all about "the buzz"—helping each child tap into his or her unique wellspring of "joy, excitement, humor, and passion," the key elements of the "creation" tenet of Gestalt therapy. The goal, he says, is to discover "how that kid *is* in the world." Academics are a critical component of that portrait: How does the child take in information? How does he express himself verbally? In writing? Is he reading at grade level? If not, does he have a learning disability? Do his behavior problems in the classroom signal a biologically based learning problem? The psychologist's day-to-day interactions with troubled kids make Hanson painfully aware of what can happen when schools neglect to identify hidden disabilities, which are often masked, ironically, by the child's obvious intelligence and creativity. He adheres to the "sea of strengths" model described in Sally Shaywitz's book *Overcoming Dyslexia*, which views dyslexia as an "encapsulated" weakness among a host of gifts, such as problem-solving and reasoning abilities, excellence in comprehension and concept formation, and well-developed general knowledge and vocabulary (58).

When bright kids struggle along for years with undiagnosed disabilities such as dyslexia, their self-concept takes a pummeling. The emotional and psychological scars inflicted by untreated learning problems are avoidable, Hanson insists, if schools detect and address them right away, preferably in kindergarten. Serving his second stint as president of the Oregon chapter of the National Association of School Psychologists in 2006–07, Hanson has made it his mission to advocate for LD prevention and early intervention, not only at MLC but throughout the district—because there's only so much Rousseau can do to help, once the damage is done.

Q: What percent of children who are identified with a disability in the Portland School District have disabilities specifically in reading?

HANSON: Our numbers are comparable to the numbers across the nation. We've seen a great increase in the number of students identified with learning disabilities, particularly in reading. Between 60 percent and 75 percent of our kids identified with a disability have a learning disability. Most of those are in reading. We're doing a better job identifying them, and the same holds true with communication disorders like autism and Asperger's syndrome. My case load has tripled in three years.

Q: How do reading disabilities affect achievement in other academic areas?

HANSON: Reading is the core skill. If you can't read by the time you get to fourth grade, you're going to start having significant difficulty across the content areas.

Q: What triggered your concerns about how and when learning disabilities are identified?

HANSON: My major concern was that we were not identifying students early enough and getting them services early enough. We know that we can do a pretty good job of identification relatively early. Certainly by age six or seven we can identify problems in the core skills involved in reading, and assess whether someone has fallen behind or has not made expected progress. That's the time to intervene. Nationally, most reading disabilities aren't identified until almost third grade. And students spend far too long in special education. Many of the kids identified with learning disabilities in third grade stay in special education until they graduate from high school. If we can identify kids earlier and get them more intense support services, we can stop that from happening.

Q: How does a too-late intervention affect the child's psychological well-being?

HANSON: Kids know early on when they're not reading like their buddies. For some kids that can be devastating. They start to avoid reading, and it turns into a vicious cycle.

Q: Research shows that kids who lag behind in third grade almost never catch up to their peers, yet many educators resist identifying reading disabilities in kindergarten or first grade. Why is that?

HANSON: Educators are trying hard to keep up with the science of the last fifteen years in reading acquisition. It takes a long time for science to come into practice. Besides, there is disagreement among researchers and also a failure of communication between researchers and practitioners. So it's often difficult, first, to develop policy for providing identification and services and, second, to make that policy comprehensive enough with full funding to be effective. Education budgets are always on the chopping block.

Q: How are you and the faculty here at MLC addressing the early-identification issue?

HANSON: Our teachers know quickly if a student is not making expected progress. They have no hesitancies in referring children. Also, we've moved toward using schoolwide screenings. We use DIBELS in kindergarten to identify kids the teacher might not pick up. We are also developing a research grant that will combine response-to-intervention strategies with what we know about the neuroscience of reading and how that science correlates with the Cattell-Horn-Carroll theory of intelligence. Essentially, that means tapping in to working memory, auditory processing, processing speed, and reading with our current standardized intellectual and academic assessment instruments. We can use these instruments in new and potentially more valid ways.

Q: Did you initiate the move to DIBELS at MLC?

HANSON: Yes. But there's also a districtwide pilot project for early identification of learning disabilities. It was launched a couple of years ago in nearly sixty schools, mostly lower SES schools and Reading First schools, to screen, intervene, gauge the response to intervention, and then go forward with the identification.

Q: How does the district stand on the three-tier model recommended by NASP?

HANSON: Our school psychologist learning-disabilities committee has endorsed the NASP three-tier model, which calls for prevention, early intervention, and a comprehensive evaluation. We need to get services to kids earlier. I think we've been ignoring Tiers 1 and 2 far too long. But we also need Tier 3—the comprehensive assessment. The third tier can help answer very specific questions about how dyslexia looks for a particular child. That being said, any time you make decisions about service delivery models that impact a lot of kids, teachers, support people, and parents, you have to have an administrative structure that supports the process. All of those things take time and money and expertise. One of my concerns is with un-funded mandates—not providing the necessary internal support structures, first, to talk about the research so people are aware of current findings and, second, to talk about how to incorporate those findings. We need a constant source of funding that we can count on.

Q: What is the most important thing that school psychologists provide for LD kids?

HANSON: We are the educational team members that teachers or parents first come to when they notice difficulties. We can certainly help in the initial identification of those kids and in helping to design and monitor interventions so that they can learn to read better. That's also an argument for making sure we have the liberty, the funds, and the time necessary to do comprehensive assessments for students. There can be a lot of factors going on for kids, and we need to take a look at all of them.

Does the student have a language, phonetic, memory access, or rapid-naming deficit? If so, what specific areas of reading are affected? We need to holistically assess students' educational environments and instruction and dynamics to really be effective.

Q: What is your top priority for the coming year?

HANSON: The most important thing is whether our state legislature adequately funds schools over the long term. It's much more effective, behaviorally and academically, to fund schools now rather than wait to deal with the effects of poverty, of violence, of crime. We know that. *That* research we've known about for a long time.

References

Abbott, S., and V. Berninger. 1999. It's never too late to remediate: A developmental approach to teaching word recognition. *Annals of Dyslexia 49* 223–250.

Adams, M. J. 1990a. Beginning reading instruction in the United States. Bloomington, Ind.: ERIC Clearinghouse on Reading and Communication Skills. ED321250.

———. 1990b. *Beginning to read: Thinking and learning about print.* Cambridge, Mass.: MIT Press.

———. 1998. The three-cueing system. In *Literacy for all: Issues in teaching and learning*, edited by J. Osborn and F. Lehr, 73–99. New York: Guilford Press.

Adams, M. J. and J. Osborn. 1990. Beginning reading instruction in the United States. Paper presented at the meeting of the Educational Policy Group, Washington, D.C., May 16, *ERIC Digest*. Bloomington, Ind.: ERIC Clearinghouse on Reading and Communication Skills. ED 320128.

Adler, J. 1998. Open minds and the argument from ignorance. *Skeptical Inquirer* 22 (1): 41–44.

Amazon.com. Webster's Third New International Dictionary. From www.amazon.com (accessed August 18, 2004).

Anderson, D. 2004. Interview by L. Sherman. Circa March 15, Portland.

Arthur, C. 2004. Interview by Ramsey, B., and L. Sherman. Oct. 13, Portland.

Association for Direct Instruction (1995–1996). Focus: What was that Project Follow Through? *Effective School Practices* 15(1).

Baker, B. 2004. Interview by Ramsey, B., and L. Sherman. July 9, Portland.

Bateman, B. 2004. Interview by Ramsey, B., and L. Sherman. Oct. 29, Creswell.

Beck, I. 1996. *Discovering reading research.* Paper presented at the Reading Hall of Fame, International Reading Association, New Orleans. April.

Beers, T. 1987. Schema-theoretic models of reading: Humanizing the machine. *Reading Research Quarterly* 22:369–77.

Berliner, D. C. 1987. Knowledge is power: A talk to teachers about a revolution in the teaching profession. In *Talks to teachers*, edited by D. C. Berliner and B. V. Rosenshine, 3–33. New York: Random House.

Berninger, V. W. 1998. *Process assessment of the learner guides for intervention: Reading and writing*. San Antonio: The Psychological Corporation, Harcourt Brace & Co.

———. 2002. Interview by Sherman, L., Circa Jan. 15, Seattle.

———. 2005. Interview by Ramsey, B., and Sherman, L. March 29, Seattle.

———. 2006. A developmental approach to learning disabilities. In *Handbook of Child Psychology*, edited by B. Damon and R. Lerner. Vol. IV, *Child Psychology and Practice*, edited by I. Siegel and A. Renninger. New York: John Wiley & Sons. 420–452.

Berninger, V. W., S. A. Stage, D. R. Smith, and D. Hildebrand. 2001. Assessment for reading and writing intervention: A three-tier model for prevention and remediation. In *Handbook of Psychoeducational Assessment* edited by J. J. W. Andrews, D. H. Saklofske, and H. L. Janzen. San Diego: Academic Press. 195–223.

Berninger, V. W., S. P. Thalberg, I. DeBruyn, and R. Smith. 1987. Preventing reading disabilities by assessing and remediating phonemic skills. *School Psychology Review* 16(4): 554–65.

Biancarosa, G., and C. E. Snow. 2004. *Reading next: A vision for action and research in middle and high school literacy: A report to Carnegie Corporation of New York*. Washington, D.C.: Alliance for Excellent Education.

Birsh, J. R., ed. 1999. *Multisensory teaching of basic language skills*. Baltimore, Md.: Paul H. Brookes.

Bloomfield, L. 1933. *Language*. New York: Holt, Rinehart & Winston.

Blumenfeld, S. L. 1999. Politics and phonics. From www.worldnetdaily.com/news/article.asp?ARTICLE_ID = 16199 (accessed June 17, 2004).

Booth, S. (ed.) 1977. *Shakespeare's sonnets*. New Haven and London: Yale University Press (Sonnet 18 originally published in 1609).

Braun, D. 2004. Interview by Ramsey, B., and L. Sherman. April 6, Eugene.

Brooks, D. 2005. Interview by Ramsey, B., and L. Sherman. Jan. 23, Portland.

Calfee, R. C., and P. A. Drum. 1978. Learning to read: Theory, research, and practice. *Curriculum Inquiry* 8(3). 183–249.

Caplan, G., and H. Grunebaum. 1967. Perspectives on primary prevention. *Archives of General Psychiatry* 17.

Carter, J. 2004. Interview by Ramsey, B., and L. Sherman. April 7, Eugene.

Chall, J. S. 1967, 1983. *Learning to read: The great debate*. New York: McGraw-Hill (updated Edition, 1983).

Chall, J. S., V. A. Jacobs, and L. E. Baldwin. 1990. *The reading crisis: Why poor children fall behind*. Cambridge, Mass.: Harvard University Press.

Coleman, J. S., E. Q. Campbell, C. J. Hobson, J. McPartland, A. M. Mood, F. D. Weinfeld, and R. L. York. 1966. *Equality of educational opportunity*. Washington, D.C.: U.S. Department of Health, Education, and Welfare, Office of Education.

Cole, C. 2004. Interview with Ramsey, B. and L. Sherman. April 6, Eugene.

Dale. 2003. Interview by Ramsey, B., and L. Sherman. Aug. 11, Pendleton.

Dewey, J. 1938. *Experience and education*. New York: Simon & Schuster.

Edelsky, C., B. Altwerger, and B. Flores. 1991. *Whole language: What's the difference?* Portsmouth, N.H.: Heinemann.

Edward de Vere Newsletter. 2001. *Dr. Knox Middle School* (Kelowna, B.C.). From http://drk.sd23.bc.ca/DeVere/Langham_Orthography-26.pdf (accessed March 16, 2006).

Ehri, L. C. 1998. Research on learning to read and spell: A personal-historical perspective. *Scientific Studies of Reading* 2(2): 97–114.

Elley, W. 1997. No cause for panic over reading levels. *New Zealand Education Review.* 10.

Fiske, E. B. 1975. About education: Approach to reading rethought. *New York Times*, July 9, 27.

Flesch, R. 1955. *Why Johnny can't read and what you can do about it.* New York: Harper & Brothers.

———. 1981. *Why Johnny still can't read.* New York: Harper & Row.

Foorman, B. R., and J. K. Torgesen. 2001. Critical elements of classroom and small-group instruction promote reading success in all children. *Learning Disabilities Research and Practice* 16(4): 203–12.

Fries, C. C. 1962. *Linguistics and reading.* New York: Holt, Rinehart, & Winston.

Frost, R. 1949. *Complete poems of Robert Frost.* New York: Henry Holt & Co. ("Design" originally published in 1936).

Gaskins, I. W., L. C. Ehri, C. Cress, C. O'Hara, and K. Donnelly. 1996–1997. Procedures for word learning: Making discoveries about words. *Reading Teacher* 50(4): 312–27.

Good, R. 2004. Interview by Ramsey, B., and L. Sherman. Oct. 29, Eugene.

Goodman, K. 1986. *What's whole in whole language: A parent/teacher guide to children's learning.* Portsmouth, N.H.: Heinemann.

———. 2002. An inquisition for school research? *Education Week* 21(22), 48.

Gopnik, A., A. Meltzoff, and P. Kuhl. 1999. *The scientist in the crib.* New York: William Morrow.

Gordon, L. 2005. Online interview with Sherman, L. (e-mail). March 10.

Groff, P. 1977. The new anti-phonics. *Elementary School Journal* 77, 323–32.

Gough, P. B., J. A. Alford, and P. Holley-Wilcox. 1981. Words and contexts. In *Perception of print: Reading research in experimental psychology*, edited by O. J. Tzeng and H. Singer. Hillsdale, N.J.: Lawrence Erlbaum Associates. 85–100.

Gove, P. B., ed. 2002. Webster's third new international dictionary of the English language, unabridged. Springfield, Mass.: Merriam-Webster.

Guckenberger vs. *Boston University*, 974 F. Supp. 106 (D. Mass., 1997).

Haigler, K. O., C. Harlow, P. O'Connor, and A. Campbell. 1994. Executive summary of literacy behind prison walls: Profiles of the prison population from the National Adult Literacy Survey. National Center for Education Statistics. From http://nces.ed.gov/naal/resources/execsummprison.asp (accessed Feb. 1, 2005).

Hall, S. L., and L. C. Moats. 1999. *Straight talk about reading: How parents can make a difference in the early years.* Chicago: Contemporary Books.

Hallahan, D. P., and C. D. Mercer. 2002 Learning disabilities: Historical perspectives. In *Identification of learning disabilities: Research to practice*, edited by R. Bradley, L. Danielson, and D. P. Hallahan, 1–67. Mahwah, N.J.: Lawrence Erlbaum.

Hanson, J. 2004. Interview by Sherman, L. June 4. Portland.

Haycock, K., and S. Huang. 2001. Are today's high school graduates ready? *Thinking K-16* 5(1). Washington, D.C.: The Education Trust. 3–17.

Hempenstall, K. 1997. The whole language-phonics controversy: An historical perspective. *Educational Psychology* 17(4). 399–418.

Hirsch, E. D., Jr. 2001. Seeking breadth and depth in the curriculum. *Educational Leadership* 59(2). 22–25.

———. 2003. General and particular aims of education. *Principal Leadership* 3(7). 20–23.

Holloway, D. 2004. Interview by Ramsey, B., and L. Sherman. Oct. 12. Portland.

Huey, E. B. 1968. *The psychology and pedagogy of reading.* Cambridge, Mass.: MIT Press. Originally published in 1908.

International Reading Association's Phonics Special Interest Group. 2003. *Phonics Bulletin* vol. 1. From www.phonicsbulletin.info/phonicsbulletin2003.pdf (accessed March 16, 2006).

Johnson, J. 2004. Interview by Sherman, L. April 7, Eugene.

Juel, C. 1988. Learning to read and write: A longitudinal study of fifty-four children from first through fourth grade. *Journal of Educational Psychology* 80:437–47.

Kame'enui, E. J., D. C. Simmons, and M. D. Coyne. 2000. Schools as host environments: Toward a schoolwide reading improvement model. *Annals of Dyslexia* 50:33–51.

Kame'enui, E. 2004. Interview by Ramsey, B., and Sherman, L. May 21, Eugene.

Kantrowitz, B., and A. Underwood. 1999. Dyslexia and the new science of reading. *Newsweek* 134(21): 72–78.

Kaplan, K. 2002. Interview by Sherman, L. Circa Nov. 15, Portland.

King, R., and J. K. Torgesen. 2000. Improving the effectiveness of reading instruction in one elementary school: A description of the process. *Florida Center for Reading Research.* FCRR Technical Report #3. From www.fcrr.org/TechnicalReports/Hartsfieldnew.pdf (accessed March 16, 2006).

Kirsch, I. S., A. Jungeblut, and L. Jenkins. 1993. *Adult literacy in America: A first look at the results of the National Adult Literacy Survey.* Washington, D.C.: National Center for Education Statistics.

Kozloff, M. A. 2002. Rhetoric and revolution: Kenneth Goodman's "psycholinguistic guessing game." *University of North Carolina, Wilmington.* From http://people.uncw.edu/kozloffm/goodman.html (accessed March 16, 2006).

Krueger, A. B. 1999. But does it work? *The New York Times,* Nov. 7.

Leppin, L. 2002. Whole language and the black arts. *Education Week* 21(24): 40–41.

Lerner, J. 2003. *Learning disabilities: Theories, diagnosis, and teaching strategies,* 9th ed. Boston: Houghton Mifflin.

Levin, H. 1966. Reading research: What, why, and for whom? *Elementary English.* ERIC Database, ED011582.

Levin, J. R., and A. M. O'Donnell. 2000. *Issues in Education: Contributions from Educational Psychology* 5.1–87.

Lyon, G. R. 1996a. Special education for students with disabilities: The future of children. *LD Online* 6(1). From www.ldonline.org/ld_indepth/general_info/future_children.html (accessed March 14, 2006).

———. 1996b. Why Johnny can't decode. *Washington Post,* October 27.

———. 1998. Why reading is not a natural process. *Educational Leadership* 55(6): 14–18.

———. 2000. *Education research and evaluation and student achievement: Quality counts.* Statement to Committee on Education and the Workforce, U.S. House of Representatives, Washington, D.C., May 4.

———. 2003. Reading disability: Why do some children have difficulty learning to read and what can be done about it? *Perspectives* 29(2): 17–19.

———. 2004. *Converging evidence: What it takes to read.* Interview with David Boulton. *Children of the Code.* From www.childrenofthecode.org/interviews/lyon.htm (accessed March 14, 2006).

Mackley, J. 2005. Interview by Ramsey, B., and L. Sherman. Jan. 10, Portland.

Manzo, K. K. 1998. Study finds distinctive brain patterns in people with dyslexia. *Education Week* 17 (26): 7.

———. 2004. Father of "whole language" rallying against reading-group speaker. *Education Week* 23(25): 11.

Martin, M. 2004. Interview by Ramsey, B., and L. Sherman. April 7, Eugene.

McDonnell, K. 2003. *Swift, Lord, you are not.* Collegeville, Minn.: St. John's University Press.

Moats, L. C. 1999. Teaching reading is rocket science: What expert teachers of reading should know and be able to do. *American Federation of Teachers*. From www.aft.org/pubs-reports/downloads/teachers/rocketsci.pdf (accessed March 14, 2006).

———. 2000. *Whole language lives on: The illusion of "balanced" instruction.* Washington, D.C.: Thomas B. Fordham Foundation.

Nagy, W. E., and R. C. Anderson. 1984. How many words are there in printed English? *Reading Research Quarterly* 19(3): 304–30.

National Association of School Psychologists. 2003. *NASP recommendations for IDEA reauthorization: Identification and eligibility determination for students with specific learning disabilities.* NASP. From www.nasponline.org/advocacy/LDRecs_042803.pdf (accessed March 14, 2006).

National Center for Education Statistics. 2003a. *National Assessment of Adult Literacy.* From http://nces.ed.gov/naal/design/about02.asp (accessed Feb. 1, 2005).

National Center for Education Statistics. 2003b. *NAEP, the Nation's Report Card.* From http://nces.ed.gov/nationsreportcard/reading/results2003/natachieve-lunch-gr4.asp (accessed April 7, 2005).

National Center for Education Statistics. 2003c. Overview of 1992 results. From http://nces.ed.gov/naal/resources/92results.asp (accessed Feb. 1, 2005).

National Endowment for the Arts. 2004. *Reading at risk: A survey of literary reading in America: Research Division Report #46.* Washington, DC: Author.

National Reading Panel: Reports of the Subgroups. 2000. *Teaching children to read: An evidence-based assessment of the scientific research literature on reading and its implications for reading instruction.* National Institutes of Health, Washington, D.C.: Government Printing Office.

Nicholson, T. 1997. Whole language goes up, reading standards go down: Fact or fiction? *School of Education, University of Auckland (New Zealand).* From www.aare.edu.au/97/pap/nicht485.htm (accessed Jan. 27, 2005).

Pearson, P. D. 1989. Reading the whole language movement. *Elementary School Journal*, 90(2). 231–41.

———. 1999. A historically based review of preventing reading difficulties in young children. *Reading Research Quarterly* 34:231–46.

———. 2001. Reading in the twentieth century. *Center for the Improvement of Early Reading Achievement.* From www.ciera.org/library/archive/2001-08/0108pdp.pdf (accessed March 14, 2006).

Pearson, P. D., and T. E. Raphael. 2003. Toward a more complex view of balance in the literacy curriculum. In *Best practices in literacy instruction*, edited by P. D. Pearson, T. E. Raphael, and M. Pressley. Guilford Press. 23–42.

Piaget, J. 1969. *Science of education and the psychology of the child.* New York: Viking Press.

Pinker, S. 1994. *The language instinct.* New York: William Morrow.

Post, A. 2004. Interview by Ramsey, B., and L. Sherman. October 15, Portland.

Routman, R. 1988. *Transitions: From Literature to Literacy.* Portsmouth, N.H.: Heinemann.

Routman, R. 1994. *Invitations: Changing as teachers and learners K-12.* Portsmouth, N.H.: Heinemann.

Rubin, H. G. 2002. Researchers link dyslexia to specific area of brain. West Palm Beach, *Education Daily.*

Ruff, J. 2004. Interview by Ramsey, B., and L. Sherman. March 22, Portland.

Sacks, O. 1995. *An anthropologist on Mars: Seven paradoxical tales.* New York: Knopf.

Schieffer, C., N. E. Marchand-Martella, R. C. Martella, F. L. Simonsen, and K. M. Waldron-Soler. 2002. An analysis of the Reading Mastery program: Effective components and research review. *Journal of Direct Instruction* 2:87–119.

Shaywitz, B. A., S. E. Shaywitz, K. R. Pugh, W. E. Mencl, R. K. Fulbright, P. Skudlarski, R. T. Constable, K. E. Marchione, J. M. Fletcher, G. R. Lyon, and J. C. Gore. (2002). Disruption of posterior brain systems for reading in children with developmental dyslexia. *Biological Psychiatry* (52), 101–110.

Shaywitz, S. 2003. *Overcoming dyslexia: A new and complete science-based program for reading problems at any level.* New York: Alfred A. Knopf.

Shlafly, P. 1999. Beware of the phonics conspiracy. *The Phyllis Shlafly Report* 33(3). From www.eagleforum.org/psr/1999/oct99/psroct99.html (accessed March 14, 2006).

Slavin, R. E., and N. Madden. 1989. What works for students at risk: A research synthesis. *Educational Leadership* 64:4–13.

Snow, C. E., S. Burns, and P. Griffin, eds. 1998. *Preventing reading difficulties in young children.* Washington, DC: National Research Council.

Spittal, C. 2004. Interview by Ramsey, B., and L. Sherman. Oct. 14, Gresham.

Spittal, K. 2004. Interview by Ramsey, B., and L. Sherman. Oct. 14, Gresham.

Stahl, S. A., J. Osborn and F. Lehr. 1990. *Beginning to read: Thinking and learning about print—A summary.* Champaign, IL: Center for the Study of Reading, University of Illinois.

Stadel, C. 2004. Interview by Lee Sherman. Nov. 3, Portland.

Stanovich, K. E. 1994. Constructionism in reading education. *Journal of Special Education* 28(3): 259–74.

Stanovich, P. J., and K. E. Stanovich. 2003. *Using research and reason in education: How teachers can use scientifically based research to make curricular and instructional decisions.* Washington, D.C.: National Institute for Literacy.

Stephenson, F. 2002. A left-right call to arms. *Research in Review* (Summer). Florida State University. From www.research.fsu.edu/researchr/summer2002/phonics/calltoarms.html (accessed June 5, 2005).

Swanson, C. 2003. Interview by Ramsey, B., and L. Sherman. August 10, Pendleton.

Terhune, A. P. 1919. *Lad: A dog.* New York: E. P. Dutton.

Tibbetts, D. 2002. Interview by Sherman, L. Circa Nov. 15, Portland.

"Tony." 2004. Interview by Sherman, L. Circa Jan. 15, Portland.

Torgesen, J. K. 1998. Catch them before they fall: Identification and assessment to prevent reading failure in young children. *American Educator* 22(1–2): 32–39.

———. 1999. Assessment and instruction for phonemic awareness and word recognition skills. In *Language and reading disabilities*, edited by H. W. Catts and A. G. Kamhi. Boston: Allyn & Bacon. 128–149.

———. 2002. The prevention of reading difficulties. *Journal of School Psychology* 40(1): 7–26

Torgesen, J. K., A. W. Alexander, R. K. Wagner, C.A. Rashotte, K. K. S. Voeller, and T. Conway. 2001. Intensive remedial instruction for children with severe reading disabilities: Immediate and long-term outcomes from two instructional approaches. *Journal of Learning Disabilities* 34(1): 33–58, 78.

Twain, M. 1884. *The adventures of Huckleberry Finn*. New York: Harper & Brothers.

University of Washington Office of News and Information. 2000. Novel treatment helps dyslexics significantly improve reading skills, shows the brain changes as children learn. May 24.

Vaughn, S., S. W. Moody, and J. S. Schumm. 1998. Broken promises: Reading instruction in the resource room. *Exceptional Children* 83(1): 211–25.

Weaver, C. 1994. *Reading process and practice: From socio-psycholinguistics to whole language*, 2nd ed. Portsmouth, N.H.: Heinemann.

Weir, R. 1990. Philosophy, cultural beliefs, and literacy. *Interchange* 21(4): 24–33.

Whitehead, D. 2004. Interview by Ramsey, B., and L. Sherman. August 7, Portland.

William. 2003. Interview by Ramsey, B., and L. Sherman. August 11, Pendleton.

Wingert, P., and B. Kantrowitz. 1997. Why Andy couldn't read. *Newsweek* 130(17): 56–64.

Wolter, R. 2004. Interview by Ramsey, B., and L. Sherman. April 6, Eugene.

Wright, J. 2004. Interview by Ramsey, B., and L. Sherman. Dec. 17, Portland.

Wyrick, C. 2004. Interview by Ramsey, B., and L. Sherman. Jan. 23, Portland.

Wyrick, E. 2004. Interview by Ramsey, B., and L. Sherman. May 22, Eugene.

Ziffer, D. 2002. Whole language and the black arts. *Education Week* 21(24): 40–41.

About the Authors

Lee Sherman is a research writer at Oregon State University. Since earning her master's degree in journalism from the University of Oregon in 1980, she has worked as a reporter, editor, and freelance writer for a number of Northwest publications. She was co-editor of *Northwest Education* magazine, published by the Northwest Regional Educational Laboratory, when it received the 1997 Golden Lamp award from the Association of Educational Publishers (EdPress) for best education magazine for an adult audience in the nation. Her work also has received recognition from the Oregon Newspaper Publishers Association, the Oregon Society of Professional Journalists, and the Alliance of Area Business Publications.

Betsy Ramsey holds degrees in biology and medical technology and works as a research associate in the Oregon Cancer Institute of Oregon Health & Science University. She currently is the coordinator of a project studying biological markers of clinical outcome in breast cancer patients. She has long been an advocate for children with learning disabilities and has served as chair of the Oregon State Advisory Council for Special Education, president of the Oregon Branch of the International Dyslexia Association, and member of the Oregon Literacy Leadership State Steering Committee. She in a member of the Board of Oregon Parent Training and Information where she volunteers in the IEP Partners Project as a coach to help parents become better informed and effective participants in the educational care of their children.